Health Secrets from Europe

Paavo O. Airola, N. D.

Foreword by
Jern Hamberg, M.D.

ARCO PUBLISHING COMPANY, INC.
219 Park Avenue South, New York, N.Y. 10003

Dedicated to

Anni, Evi, Paul, Karen and Paula
with fatherly love
and a hopeful wish
that the application of the information presented herein
will enable them to enjoy long, happy lives
in vibrant health and perpetual youth.

Seventh Printing, 1978

An ARC Book
Published by Arco Publishing Co., Inc.
219 Park Avenue South, New York, N.Y. 10003
by arrangement with Parker Publishing Co., Inc.

Library of Congress Catalog Card Number 79-135618

ISBN 0-668-02411-9

Printed in the United States of America

Foreword by a Doctor of Medicine

The art of healing, through centuries of effort by dedicated researchers and talented scientists, has developed into today's highly esteemed and respected science of medicine—as a result, the lives of millions of people have been saved. Man now enjoys relative medical security—and the deserving researchers have been honored and given medals and prizes by a grateful humanity.

But medals have two sides. Although medical security has increased, our lives are still in great danger. In spite of a high living standard, our health standards are incredibly low. Increased prosperity seems to go hand in hand with the increased number of crimes, misuse of alcohol and drugs, moral degeneration, chronic and degenerative diseases—and more unhappiness and discontentment, generally. Modern man must have the skill of a tight-rope artist in order to retain his health, happiness and sense of balance in the busy, competitive world, which he has created for himself. Why? Because the false ideals and distorted values, the "Keeping up with the Joneses" in competition for greater material wealth, prestige, and social importance, are tapping man's lifeblood, throwing him out of balance, and undermining his health, physically as well as mentally. Disease is the logical consequence of this lost sense of values and general disharmony in modern man's life.

How does our highly developed medical science help man in his precarious condition? Does it help him to retain a balance and harmony with his environment and encourage him to take preventive measures in respect to his health? Regretfully, we have to admit that instead of encouraging positive *health-thinking*, we lure man into passive *disease-thinking*. "Why worry about health? Let me enjoy eating, drinking and living the way I like. If I get sick, the doctor will fix me up: penicillin will take care of the fever; pain tablets will remove the headache; laxatives restore regularity; tranquilizers take care of my anxieties and worries. . . ." Man has an almost superstitious faith in medical science and "wonder drugs." This passive dependence leads his attention away from the highest

7

form of medicine, *preventive medicine*, which is characterized by an active, do-it-yourself health-building effort.

It can be said that disease is a result of an unfit, improper environment and/or a faulty mode of living—an imbalance and disharmony. The doctor's aim must be to teach man a healthier way of living and help him to achieve a better biological environment—for his body as well as for his soul. The doctor himself must be a good example of the product he sells—*health*. Man should be encouraged to build up his resistance and prevent disease by a health-promoting way of life under the doctor's guidance.

It is with great joy and interest that I have read this book. Its importance for diseased mankind cannot be overestimated. It will not suit or please everyone—but what book does? If you are willing to sacrifice some time and effort to regain or improve your health, this book can offer you a large arsenal of helpful advice which will enable you to accomplish a worthwhile end.

I am personally familiar with most of the clinics mentioned in the various chapters of this book. I have studied the biological methods described and have a firsthand experience in their effectiveness, especially in the prevention of disease. Unfortunately, not all patients follow the advice given by the biologically-oriented doctors, the advice so richly contained in this book. Man chooses to follow the law of lesser resistance—and therefore pays with suffering and disease for the violation of the health laws of Nature. Those who earnestly search for better health, must change from passive disease-thinking into an active *health thinking*. This book will show you the way. It will be of great value to those who are willing to put forth the effort.

The road to better health may not always be easy. Determination and persistence are required to follow this path. This is why so many choose to passively follow the wider road that leads to disease. You must choose the narrow way if you wish to conquer disease and build better health.

The author of this book has an extraordinary dedication and ability to help you on your way to good health. The road to better health is marked by several milestones. You will learn much about these milestones to better health when you read this book. If you will wisely choose to follow the author's competent advice, your rewards will be many—better health, a greater physical and mental efficiency, and a happier state of mind.

—*Jern Hamberg, M.D.*

What This Book Can Do for You

Your probable reaction to the title of this book was: Why Europe? What possibly can we learn from Europe in the matters of health and longevity? This book will show you that we can learn a great deal.

First, while Americans are basically cure-minded, Europeans are prevention-minded. Our research in such vital fields as cancer, arthritis, cardiovascular diseases, diabetes, multiple sclerosis, etc., has been directed towards discovery of some chemical agent, a drug, which will cure or control the disease. Much of European research is directed toward the discovery of the *causative factors of disease* and developing means of preventing it.

Second, and perhaps the most important fact, is that in the United States, we largely ignore nutrition as the possible causative as well as a preventive and curative factor in disease. Europeans, on the other hand, have been much more open-minded and unprejudiced in this respect. In this book I will show how many of our common health problems can be solved by improved nutrition. Arthritis, prostate problems, colds, high blood pressure, multiple sclerosis, ulcers, psoriasis, miscarriages, heart disease—these are just a few of the diseases European doctors treat with dietetic restrictions and vitamin-mineral therapies.

This book brings to you much needed health information in the form of easy-to-follow, do-it-yourself instructions based on European studies and experiences, which will help you to improve your health, increase your vitality and prolong your life.

In the following chapters you will learn:

- How you can increase your vitality and avoid unnecessary degenerative diseases with the world-famous Waerland health system.
- How arthritis is cured in European clinics by biological therapies.
- How environmental and nutritional therapies developed in Germany and Russia fight one of man's most dreadful killers, heart disease, and how these therapies are helping millions of people in European health reconditioning centers.
- How multiple sclerosis is cured in Europe by nutritional means.

- How, with simple changes in your nutritional habits, you can help prevent premature aging and start looking years younger than your calendar age.
- How European biological clinics and health spas use various water cures, fasts, overheating therapies, and other unconventional methods and special foods to cure many of our most commón ailments.
- How you can revitalize your sex life by feeding your glands more effectively.
- How prostate disorders can be prevented or corrected by nutritional means.
- How latest European discoveries can help you to grow hair.
- How you can keep younger longer with wonder-foods from the bees: pollen, royal jelly and honey.
- How to prepare and use special health and longevity foods from Europe.

I have a firsthand experience and knowledge of what I am writing about. I have visited clinics and·research institutions, and have interviewed doctors and patients in Germany, Sweden, Switzerland, Russia, and many other countries. I have studied the records and checked the case histories. The case histories presented in this book are all actual cases, gathered and checked by me personally, or taken from reputable publications. Each chapter on European health methods and biological therapies is supplemented by detailed do-it-yourself instructions adapted to American conditions. Recipes and directions for the unusual European health-giving longevity foods are supplied in the last chapter.

It is my conviction that if you read this book with an open and unprejudiced mind and follow the outlined programs, you will be rewarded with improved health and a longer, happier life.

Your health is your most precious possession. Your efforts to learn the secrets of preserving health and avoiding sickness will be repaid with rich dividends. Let me be your guide on an exciting journey to better health and longer life—the European way!

—*Paavo O. Airola, N.D.*

Table of Contents

Health Secrets from Europe

1

What Americans Can Learn from Europe about Better Health

In spite of the great medical progress and the billions of dollars spent on health care in the United States today, it is estimated that there are still in this country over 80 million chronically ill people. The most distressing fact is that instead of improving, the situation is worsening with every passing year. There is an epidemic increase in such diseases as heart disease, cancer, arthritis, allergies, multiple sclerosis, and birth defects. Our mortality rate is higher than in most civilized countries; and in life expectancy among nations, the United States ranks 22nd for men and 10th for women. Many responsible scientists have expressed their concern and called the health conditions of this nation *"catastrophic."*

What are the reasons for such an appalling and frightful deterioration of the health of the American people? The main reason for this is our artificial, sedentary, air-conditioned way of life in a denatured, synthetic, chemicalized, and poisoned environment. *Nutrition is the most important single environmental factor affecting one's health.* But, according to a recent U.S. Department of Agriculture survey, only half of the American households are found to be eating a nutritionally adequate diet. The other half of the American people are *malnourished.*

Why, in the country that has the most abundant supply of food in the world, should one half of the population be malnourished?

The answer is: because of ignorance. "People just don't know what kinds of foods are necessary for good health and vigor," said Assistant Secretary of Agriculture, George L. Mehren. The nutrition Americans obtain today in the form of devitalized, factory-produced and chemicalized food, loaded with poisonous residues from additives and pesticides, can result only in deteriorated health. Add to this the air poisoned with deadly chemicals, the polluted water, and the gigantic consumption of toxic drugs, and you will have found most of the reasons for the appalling deterioration of our health.

The extensive and prolonged use of chemical fertilizers has depleted our soils and, although the quantity of the crops still remains high with the help of constantly increasing amounts of chemical fertilizers, *the nutritional quality of foods produced on depleted soils is lowered.* For example, wheat grown in the American midwest in the beginning of the century contained an average 17–18 percent of protein; sometimes it even went as high as over 20 percent. Now, the average content of protein in our wheat is only 12–14 percent, often even less. Just imagine what this significant difference in the content of one of the most important nutritional elements will do to your health! In Russia, wheat still contains 16–18 percent protein. Professor Barry Commoner, of Washington University in St. Louis, said that a slice of American bread needs a slice of cheese on it to match the slice of plain Russian bread in nutritional value!

The mineral and vitamin content of processed foods produced on depleted soils with the help of chemical fertilizers is equally reduced. For example, nutritionist Dr. H. K. Stieberling writes in the *Journal of the American Dietetic Association* that the *national food supply is about 15 percent lower in vitamins A and C today than it was 20 years ago.*

Continuous and widespread use of poisonous insecticides in production, processing and handling of foodstuffs has resulted in greater and greater residues of them in foods.

In addition to pesticides, foods are loaded with various other toxic chemicals added to it during processing. These are: preservatives, dyes, bleaches, conditioners, hydrogenators, softeners, moisteners, acidifiers, alkilizers, antioxidents, emulcifiers, and many more. Many of these are harmful and unfit for human consumption.

The air in most of our larger cities is so polluted by the poisonous gases from automobiles and industries that it is also a major health hazard. It is considered to be one of the leading causes of cancer in the respiratory organs. Emphysema, which spreads as a plague around the whole nation, is directly linked to polluted air and smoking.

Our water is just as unfit for drinking as our air is for breathing. Almost half of the American public is drinking fluoridated water in spite of the mounting evidence that the toxic effect of sodium fluoride is *one* of the reasons for the catastrophic deterioration of the health of Americans.[1]

In addition to all this, we poison ourselves in a hundred other ways in our everyday living with household chemicals, detergents, insecticides for homes and gardens, insect repellents, air-fresheners, disinfectants, hair sprays, etc. Many other things in our environment, such as clothing, rugs, wallpapers, upholstery, and mattresses, are treated with toxic chemicals.

POISONED FOOD AND ENVIRONMENT
SPELLS DISEASE AND DEATH

What do all these poisons in our food and environment do to our health? This whole book could be filled with reputable scientific evidence, facts, results of research, and actual cases to prove that poisons in our food and our environment do, indeed, harm us, make us sick, and may even kill us. Many excellent books are written on this subject; *Silent Spring* by Rachel Carson, for example.

But let me give you just a very short illustration of this point. Here is a case which is so typical in our poisoned way of life that it is happening every day—without our suspecting the real cause of the problem: In Chicago, a nine-year-old girl died after doctors could not diagnose her illness. They treated her for hypoglycemia, acidosis, and other things, without success. Finally her parents remembered that just before her acute illness the girl's bedroom was sprayed with insecticide containing chlordane and organic phosphates!

Pesticides are suspected of being one of the causes of the sharp increase in birth defects.[2] Measurable amounts of pesticides have been found in the tissues of stillborn babies. Lengthy exposure to pesticides in homes and farms can cause the fatal blood diseases, leukemia and aplastic anemia, reported a Mayo Clinic consultant Dr. M. M. Hargraves. The sharp increase in hepatitis in the U.S. may be due to wide use of insecticides.[3]

---

[1] All footnote references, beginning with number 1 and numbered consecutively throughout each chapter, are listed in a separate section at the end of this book.

Analysis of samples of foods served in restaurants showed that each food was contaminated with DDT. There are dozens of various pesticides in use in food production, and although little is known of the effect of one pesticide in combination with another, it is known that the toxic effect due to combination can be increased from 10 to 50 times!

WHAT CURE-MINDED AMERICANS CAN LEARN FROM PREVENTION-MINDED EUROPEANS

If an American shows an unusual interest and concern for his health, and especially if he dares go so far as to exercise regularly and eat health foods, he is looked upon as an odd-ball and a health-nut. In the United States, health-conscious individuals are often ridiculed and sneered at. In Europe it is the other way around. Those who try to improve their mode of living, adhere to health-promoting habits, control their eating, exercise, visit health spas, etc., are considered very smart. They are looked upon as enlightened individuals with character, conviction and wisdom. For several years now I have been living half of the year in the United States and the other half in Europe, so I speak of this from first-hand experience.

We are basically cure-minded. We don't worry about our health until we get sick. Then we go to our doctor and expect him to fix us up. Europeans are, vice versa, prevention minded—they are concerned about preserving their health and preventing disease by their own effort.

This difference in attitude is reflected also in the official policies and actions of respective governments and medical organizations. American medical research is basically directed at finding a cure, preferably with a drug, vaccine or surgery. European medical research is to a large degree directed towards the discovery of the causes of diseases, finding ways of preventing them, and then teaching these preventive ways to the public.

For example, in Germany and Russia there are over 3,000 cardiac reconditioning health centers where a person can have his health rebuilt or his heart condition corrected, and where he is instructed to follow a special regimen and diet upon his return home in order to prevent recurrence. In Russia alone it is estimated that about five million people visit such health reconditioning centers each year. In Russia, of course, all this is financed by the government, but in Germany the private industry and insurance companies have spent lavish amounts of money in setting up such centers. Dr. Peter Beckman, director of Ohlstadt Cardiac Reconditioning Center in Bavaria, tells that his program of exercise, diet and mental relaxation helps the heart patient to rebuild his health. Most of his patients are likely candidates for heart attacks, executives in their early 40's, sent there by their business or insurance companies for free preventive care.

Protection from poisons in food and environment

In regard to the threat of poison in foods and environment, European doctors and governments have demonstrated their willingness to protect the public. For example, long before Americans even heard of the possible link between smoking and cancer, several European governments, convinced by the overwhelming evidence, took action against smoking. In England tobacco advertising is under rigid restriction. In Italy it is totally banned. Heavy taxes were put on cigarettes by many countries to make them less attractive; a pack of cigarettes in Sweden, for example, costs about three times the American price!

Fluoridation of the water is another good example. Many European countries do not want anything to do with fluoridation. The government of Denmark, on recommendation of their Medical Association, totally prohibited the fluoridation of water throughout the country. Russia and many East European countries did the same. Their reason for prohibition is that "there is no valid scientific evidence as to the benefit or the harmfulness of the measure."

The scientific council of the International Society for Research on Nutrition and Vital Substances, a foremost scientific body of over 400 scientists from all over the world, has condemned fluoridation of the water. Their resolution on prevention of dental diseases states: "A diet of natural, whole foods rich in vital substances stimulating mastication should be preferred to a compulsory fluoridation of drinking water."

Where poisonous pesticides and food additives are concerned, many European countries have taken drastic measures to protect the public.

In Germany, since 1959, there has been a very strict law regulating additives to foods of *fremdestoffe* (foreign substances), implying that they don't really belong in foods. Amounts of additives permitted in foods are sharply reduced and all additives must be clearly declared, even in restaurants, where food additives used in every item on the menu must be indicated.

In France, bleached flour is not permitted to be used in bread, nor are chemical additives permitted in bread. In England, there is a government law, the Carcinogenic Substances Regulation, termed "a landmark in cancer prevention," which supervises and regulates the presence of cancer-causing chemicals in man's environment. Spain and Israel have reduced by law the chemical treatment of their fruits. And in Soviet Russia, food processors and manufacturers are not allowed to use any artificial colors or flavors in any foods whatsoever.

While we ridicule those who try to improve their health and prevent disease by eating health foods, in Sweden, top nutritionists at the famous Nobel Institute have started extensive research aimed at the development of a health-food diet that will prevent illness and build optimum health.

AN OUNCE OF PREVENTION
IS WORTH A POUND OF CURE

Here are a few examples of how the preventive approach has helped people in Europe to improve their health and prevent sickness.

At a German bathing spa I met a stout-looking executive, Mr. H.B. He is a director of one of the important industries in Hamburg. About ten years ago his doctors discovered that he had hypertension. After an unsuccessful attempt to control his high blood pressure with drugs, they sent Mr. H.B. to this famous watering spa.

"I have been coming here every summer for a week or two ever since," Mr. H.B. told me. "My pressure usually goes down to normal during this time and I feel like a new man—twenty years younger. After a winter at my work, my blood pressure rises again, so I come back here, and all these baths, relaxation and good food put me back on my feet again." Instead of endangering his life with powerful drugs, Mr. H.B. was controlling his blood pressure and restoring his health with three ancient—but not forgotten!—methods of preventive medicine: *water cure, diet,* and *relaxation.*

In Sweden, I have witnessed an excellent example of the value of preventive medicine in action. Visiting a dentist who had a family of four children, I was amazed at how healthy the children looked and especially at their beautiful white teeth. Dr. L. explained to me that the whole family was living on the so-called Waerland-diet, a lacto-vegetarian program designed by the Swedish nutritionist and health pioneer, Are Waerland. The children were raised on this program from birth. (The Waerland program is described in detail in Chapter 5). None of the children have had so much as a single cavity, although the eldest boy was already 17 years old. Knowing that this was a dentist's family, I inquired if they did lots of toothbrushing.

"Never," was Dr. L.'s answer. "I do not believe in toothbrushing. They rinse their teeth after meals, occasionally use toothpicks, and finish the meal with raw fruits or vegetables." Needless to say, white sugar, white bread, and candies can never be found in this prevention-conscious family.

Russian and German reconditioning centers have demonstrated that diseases and physical deterioration can be prevented on a large scale by proper preventive means. Millions of people, perhaps as many as eight to ten million people in these two countries alone, visit spas and reconditioning centers each year, where their health is rebuilt and future illnesses prevented by programs of exercise, diet, and mental relaxation. Thousands of potential heart attacks are prevented in these centers. In one of the German cardiac centers I met a group of 60- to 80-year-old men who have been serious heart cases for 10 to 20 years. They visit this center for six weeks each year, and they told me that their condition is improved colossally during the six weeks of Spa treatment. "These mineral waters keep me alive," an 84-year-old man, who has been coming here for the last 15 years, told me.

In the United States, we are basically cure-minded, and preventive medicine, in the sense described above, is a largely unknown occurrence here. While German industries send their executives to reconditioning health centers regularly, our economic system, with its chronic unemployment, does not favor the preventive approach. An executive who succumbs in his high-pressure job to a heart attack can be easily replaced. The rampant growth of heart diseases in the United States can be at least in part due to our neglect to take advantage of the European experience with the preventive cardiac programs.

We are still a great nation, with unmatched technological competence and a great capacity for scientific advancement. But if our economic, diplomatic, and military strength is not matched and backed up by the physical and moral stamina of our people, we may find the wheels of destiny turning to our disadvantage. Human history shows that *decay from within* in the form of physical and moral degeneration has brought about the fall of great nations. It is disheartening to witness the catastrophic health degeneration of our nation, *when the scientific knowledge of how to build and guard health and prevent sickness is available.*

A U.S. senator, concerned with the health of American people, once said that we are spending about $50 billion a year *on health.* I would like to make an important correction: virtually all of this money is spent *on disease,* not on health. If the American government would start spending money *on health and the prevention of disease,* the trend toward the rapid deterioration of the health of this nation would soon be reversed.

Meanwhile, waiting for our government's action in this respect, why not benefit from the application of some of the preventive and therapeutic methods, used successfully in Europe, which are described in the following chapters of this book?

2

Fasting — European Way
to Health and Long Life

Of all the health secrets from Europe which this book will reveal to you, fasting is, perhaps, the most valuable one from the point of your own health potential. Of course, you understand that there are no *secrets* of health or longevity in Europe or anywhere else. When we speak of health secrets from Europe we mean methods or therapies which are well-known, popular and widely practiced in Europe but hardly known or totally unrecognized in the United States. Fasting is one such "secret."

MEDICAL DOCTORS PRESCRIBE FASTING IN EUROPE

Official American medicine does not recognize fasting as one of the legitimate forms of therapy. In Europe the situation is quite different. Fasting is employed there on a grand scale by reputable medical doctors. For example, at the famous Buchinger Sanatorium in Bad Pyrmont, Germany, directed by Otto H. F. Buchinger, M.D. (perhaps the world's greatest authority on fasting), fasting is used routinely in almost every condition. Well over 70,000 fasts were supervised by medical doctors at Buchinger Clinics alone during 48 years of practice.

Another great fast specialist in Germany is Professor Werner

27

Zabel, M.D. In several decades he has used fasting as one of the most valuable therapeutic methods in his clinic for internal diseases in Berchtesgaden, Germany. "Together with fever and optimal nutrition, fasting is man's oldest healing method," said Professor Zabel.

Karolinska Institute in Stockholm, a world-famous medical research institution, has made experiments with fasting. Fasts up to 55 days were employed in their experiments. In Germany and Sweden, there are dozens of fasting clinics where fasting is an exclusive or the most important therapeutic measure.

These are only a few examples to show you that fasting in Europe is a respected and accepted form of therapy.

SWEDEN—THE PROMISED LAND OF FASTING

In Sweden fasting is used not only in the hospitals and clinics by medical practitioners, but also by thousands of health enthusiasts around the country as a positive health measure to improve health and prevent disease.

Here are a few headlines from the clippings of Swedish magazines and newspapers lying on my table:

- "Fast for better spring condition!"
- "Fast this summer to keep in shape!"
- "Eleven fasting vikings walk from Gothenburg to Stockholm (300 miles) without food!"
- "Without food for 143 days!"

Every spring and summer several groups of Swedish health enthusiasts and hundreds of individuals fast for one, two or more weeks. This is done not for the cure of any particular pathological condition, but as a kind of spring cleaning to purify their bodies from the toxins and the waste matter accumulated during long winter months of sedentary life and the lack of fresh foods. In addition, many Swedes take a regular Fasting Cure at the various biological clinics in the country under expert supervision.

FAMOUS SWEDISH FAST MARCHES

In 1954 Sweden made headlines in the world press when eleven men walked from Gothenburg to Stockholm, a distance of about 300 miles, in ten days. During the whole march these men, who walked about 30 miles each day in rain or shine, did not eat any food at all!

They didn't drink any juices, did not take any drugs, tablets or vitamins—nothing but plain water!

This fast march created a sensation not only in Sweden but around the world. Not only the average man but even the medical doctors did not realize that man can go without food for ten days, especially under such a severe physical stress. Many have heard stories of flyers who crash-landed their airplanes in the wilderness then died from starvation after eight or nine days; or of the lost mountain climbers who were starved to death after a few days. This dramatic fast march was the shock that forced people to re-assess their thinking about fasting. It made them realize that man not only can be without food for ten days but he can even perform a physical feat which many would not be able to duplicate on a diet of fat steaks.

The Gothenburg-Stockholm march received unprecedented world publicity right from the beginning. The world was not prepared for anything of this nature. Several doctors expressed their opinion that fasters would never reach Stockholm—they would die on the road. Large headlines in all the newspapers talked about "insane, mad, crack-brained faddists." Doctors suggested stopping the project by force. Sweden's largest newspaper sent a medical doctor, a specialist in athletics and sports, to check the condition of the fasters after about five days of march. Disappointed by the fact that he could not find anything wrong with the seemingly healthy and happy men, the doctor made his now infamous statement: "They remind me of a man who jumped from a skyscraper and while passing the tenth floor said to himself 'Well, so far the flight is great!' "

Hundreds of thousands of people greeted the 11 men when they triumphantly marched into Stockholm. Medical check-ups, immediately after the march, several weeks and then several months later, showed that the men did not suffer any damage. Their weight loss was an average of 20 pounds per person, or two pounds a day.

Dr. Lennart Edrén leads the fast marches

The initiative for the 1954 fast march came from Lennart Edrén, D.D.S., who was the leader and the participant in this and many subsequent fasts in Sweden. Dr. Edrén is the leading spirit behind the Swedish fast movement. Asked what was the purpose with this dramatic exhibition, Dr. Edrén said:

This fast was the first in the series of experiments to determine the effects of total fasting under severe conditions of stress. If we find out that fasting will not cause any damage to the body but will, on the contrary, exert a beneficial, revitalizing, cleansing and regenerating effect on bodily functions, it will supply invaluable information for healthy as well as for sick people. The healthy will be encouraged to fast in order to regenerate and increase vitality, and the sick to cure their ills. This experiment has proved to the world the preventive and therapeutic potentials of fasting. It also may prove very valuable for armed forces and various expeditions where the possibility of getting lost and isolated, and forced into an involuntary fast, is great.

NEW FAST MARCH IN 1964

Exactly ten years later, in August 1964, Dr. Lennart Edrén organized a second 300-mile fast march. This time there were 19 participants. While in 1954 all the participants were vegetarians with many years of healthful living and many previous experiences with fasting behind them, the 1964 group was deliberately put together of more varied types; there were vegetarians as well as meat-eaters, smokers and non-smokers, fat men and thin men, etc. In addition, the strict condition of 1954 that all must be in perfect health was not enforced in 1964. Furthermore, the 1954 fasting was a strict water fast, while in 1964 the participants received a small amount of juices in addition to water. All these changes were made with the specific purpose of making the experiment more comprehensive and scientific.

Whereas in 1954 official medicine took the position of disinterest and disapproval, the situation in 1964 was totally reversed. The whole experiment was extensively controlled and supervised by a large staff of doctors. First, all participants were given a thorough examination and various tests. Not less than five doctors were present at the start to make the final checkup. During the entire march of ten days, doctors followed the group and made daily controls and tests on the participants. This was truly a scientific experiment under the most scrupulous and careful control.

"Man's oldest therapy" wins new triumph

The 1964 fast march was a new great success. It broke the last remnants of opposition.

Karl-Otto Aly, M.D. one of the leading biologically-oriented doctors in Sweden and one of the 19 participants in the fast march, sums up the 1964 fasting as follows:

First, the march was an indisputable success and all 19 came to the finish line. Although a few had some trouble with pre-existing diseased conditions and were transported part of the distance, none interrupted their fasting. Fourteen of the 19 walked the entire 300 miles. The march clearly showed that man can live for an extended period of time without food, and can even accomplish hard physical effort while fasting. The results of all the medical tests taken before, during and after the march, have demonstrated that there are large potential reserves of strength in our bodies on which we can depend, especially under conditions of disease, when the organism usually gives indication by lack of appetite that it does not require any food. The blood pressure tests, blood serum readings, blood sugar tests, microscopic readings of uric sediment, electrocardiograms—all showed that there was no great change from the usual, and certainly no pathological developments because of fasting. This in spite of the fact that fasting was performed under such a severe stress. Perhaps it is worth noting that the overall tests of the health condition were somewhat better in 1964—with the addition of juices—than in 1954 on a pure water fast.

The most interesting observation was that the protein level (serum albumin reading) of the blood *remained constant and normal during the whole period of fasting* in spite of the fact that no protein was consumed for ten days.

Even more remarkable were the blood sugar readings. In spite of the great demands on immediate energy, and an only insignificant supply of sugar in approximately one pint of juice each day, *the sugar content of the blood remained within the normal limits.* Note that during the 1954 pure water fast the blood sugar levels remained normal, too! Thus, there were no grounds for the predicted risk of possible hypoglycemia, or pathologically low blood sugar level. Quite to the contrary, the general tendency was somewhat higher blood sugar levels after the fast than before it. Something for scientists to think about!

The generally-expressed feeling among the participants was that they felt stronger and had more vigor and vitality after the fast than before it.

The prime goal of these experiments was to stimulate scientific institutions to engage in a thorough and objective scientific study of fasting and its prophylactic and therapeutic potentials so that fasting will be generally incorporated into the growing arsenal of medical practice for the benefit and blessing to disease-ridden mankind.

WHAT IS FASTING?

Fasting is a total abstinence from food. It is the oldest therapeutic method known to man. It has been a dependable curative measure throughout medical history, even before Hippocrates, the

Father of Medicine. It was prescribed by Hippocrates, Paracelsus, Galen, and all the other great physicians of old. It was practiced by many great thinkers and philosophers, such as Plato and Socrates, to "attain mental and physical efficiency." The therapeutic values of fasting are well documented by a large number of scientific investigations, studies, and empirical observations. Doctors who employ fasting testify that it indeed works. Not only the great Paracelsus knew that "fasting is the greatest remedy," or the "physician within," but many modern medicos agree with the words of Dr. Adolph Mayer that "fasting is the most efficient means of correcting any disease." Dr. Otto H. F. Buchinger calls fasting a "Royal road to healing."

But how can mere abstinence from food accomplish such remarkable healing results?

WHY FASTING IS SO EFFECTIVE

Let me quote from my book, *There Is a Cure for Arthritis:*[1]

The therapeutic value of fasting is based on the following physiological facts:

1. Autolysis is a known metabolic phenomenon of self-digestion or disintegration of the body's own tissues.

2. Therapeutic fasting induces the development of autolysis and directs its physiological effect for constructive healing purposes.

To clarify: when disease takes hold of the body it is usually because of the weakened defensive mechanism and impaired normal functions of the vital organs. Due to continuous neglect in feeding the body properly and failure to observe the other rules of health, the glandular activity and metabolic rate slows down and the eliminative organs lose their efficiency. Many of the toxins and metabolic wastes remain in the body and are deposited in the tissues, causing autointoxication.

Now, we must recognize the fact that the body's own healing powers are constantly trying to correct any and all defects, disturbances, and damages if given the slightest chance. Such an opportunity for self-regeneration and healing is made possible during the fast.

First, during prolonged fast (after the first three days) the body will burn and digest its own tissues by the process of autolysis, or self-digestion. In its wisdom—and here lies the secret of the extraordinary effectiveness of fasting as curative therapy!—*the body will decompose and burn only those substances and tissues which are diseased, damaged, or of lesser importance to the body economy,* such as all morbid accumulations, tumors, abscesses, damaged tissues, fat deposits, etc. In fasting, the body metabolizes the most impure or inferior materials. These are consumed and utilized first. The essential tissues of vital organs are spared. Dr. Otto H. F. Buchinger calls fasting a "refuse disposal" or "burning of rubbish."

Second, the eliminating and cleansing capacity of the eliminative organs—lungs, liver, kidneys, and skin—is increased during fasting, and masses of accumulated metabolic wastes and toxins are quickly expelled. This is evident in the following typical symptoms of fasting: offensive breath, dark urine (concentration of toxins in urine ten times higher than normal [Professor E. G. Schonk]),[2] continuous and generous discharge of feces, skin eruptions, perspiration, catarrhal elimination, etc.

Third, a fast affords a physiological rest to the digestive and protective organs of the body. After fasting, the digestion and utilization of food are greatly improved, which makes the assimilation of all the important nutrients more effective.

Fourth, a fast exerts a normalizing and stabilizing effect on all the physiological, nervous, and mental functions. The nervous system is regenerated; mental powers improved; glandular chemistry and secretions are normalized.

It is easy to see from the above why fasting is such an effective healing measure in the treatment of a great variety of diseases.

HOW SAFE IS FASTING?

Earlier in the chapter you have seen some examples of how safe fasting is. Swedish fast marches have certainly proven very dramatically the safety of fasting.

Although fasting is without doubt one of the safest healing agents known to medicine, in the minds of the uninitiated and uninformed it is often associated with the fear of doing harm to the body, or even with the fear of death. Notwithstanding the fact that nobody ever died as a result of a few weeks of intentional fasting, such fears are quite understandable.

The truth is that you can live without food for months! As a matter of fact, you can more easily kill yourself by overeating than by fasting.

REAL CASES OF PROLONGED FASTING—UP TO 249 DAYS!

Recently 27-year-old Risto Lana, a Swedish philosophy student at the University of Gothenburg, fasted alternately on water and juices for a total of 143 days. No, it wasn't an anti-Vietnam demonstration; it was just an experiment for his own illumination and benefit. He lost about 60 pounds and claimed improved health, both physically and mentally, as a result of this fast.

There are recorded cases of fasting on water for up to 90 days, and up to 249 days on juices and liquids! In recent tests at the Stobhill General Hospital, in Glasgow, Scotland, a 54-year-old woman was put on a liquid fasting and lost 74 of her 262 pounds, along with a painful arthritic knee condition, during a fast of 249 days. To my knowledge, this is the longest controlled therapeutic fasting in medical history. Usually fasting is of no longer duration than 40 days, and the great majority of fasts in European clinics are only 7, 14 or 21 days long.

Naturally, if you are suffering from a serious condition such as cancer, tuberculosis, diabetes, or cardio-vascular disorders, you should be at all times under a doctor's supervision. But otherwise fasting, particularly a juice fasting, can be safely undertaken by anyone. I myself have fasted countless times and have supervised many fasts, and I can testify that fasting not only works, but is indeed one of the safest healing methods there is.

JUICE FASTING

The classic form of fasting is a pure water fast—the abstinence of all foods or drinks with the exception of pure water. However, the most common fasting method in Europe now is a so-called juice fasting. All European practitioners whom I talked with in various clinics, including the champion of therapeutic fasting in modern times, Dr. Otto H. F. Buchinger, Jr., use fresh juices of fruits and vegetables and vegetable broths and herb teas during fasting.

The medical justification of juice fasting is that freshly pressed vegetable and fruit juices will aid the patient in his recovery from disease. This is attributed to the following physiological facts:

• Raw juices, as well as freshly made vegetable broths, are rich in vitamins, minerals, trace elements and enzymes.

- These vital elements are very easily assimilated directly into the blood stream, without putting a strain on the digestive organs.
- They are extremely beneficial in normalizing the bodily processes, supplying needed elements for the body's own healing activity and thus speeding up the recovery.
- Raw juices and vegetable broths provide an alkaline surplus which is extremely important for the proper acid-alkaline balance, since blood and tissues contain large amounts of acids during fasting.

HOW FASTING CAN BE UNDERTAKEN AT HOME

Notwithstanding the fact that liquid or juice fasting is not dangerous and could be safely undertaken without supervision at home, I would advise the average person, who does not have a thorough understanding of all the phases and details of fasting, to have his fast supervised by an experienced practitioner. This will assure him peace of mind and confidence in the treatment, which are imperative for the successful outcome of any therapeutic measures.

In Sweden, of course, fasting is a national sport. Thousands of Swedes, young and old, men and women, especially the members of the Swedish health organization Hälsofrämjandet (Health Promotion) fast for a week or two almost every year. These short fasts are considered to be an effective way to cleanse the body of wastes, build up resistance and physical stamina, and prevent illness. Contrary to the popular notion, *you are not weakened or depleted by fasting*—the opposite is true. The objective which induces thousands of Swedes to fast is the total regeneration and rejuvenation of all the functions of the body. These fasts in Sweden are done by individuals in their own homes, and without the supervision of doctors, although many who suffer from various ailments do travel to biological clinics where their fasting is performed under expert supervision.

DETAILED PROGRAM FOR DO-IT-YOURSELF FASTING

Here is a short description of the mechanics of juice fasting:

First, it is advisable to prepare yourself for fasting by a short cleansing diet. For two or three days before fasting eat only raw fruits and vegetables, alternating one meal made up of any available fruits with a meal of vegetables.

On the day before the fast take a dose of castor oil in the early afternoon to clean the bowels, and do not eat any dinner. Before going to bed take a double enema. First, take one pint of plain water at body temperature, and let it out. Then repeat with a full quart. If you can make camomile tea and mix it with water, so much the better. Camomile can be obtained at drug stores or health food stores. Enemas during fasting are very important. They help the body in the elimination of toxins and waste matter from the colon and lower bowels—and you will be amazed at the amount of waste coming out with the enema even after two or three weeks of fasting!

The next day, and each following day of the fast, you follow this program:

UPON ARISING:	Cup of herb tea—lukewarm, not hot. Health food stores usually have a large assortment of herb teas. Use instructions on the package for preparing them. Peppermint, camomile, rose hips, and red clover are some of the teas which can be used.
9:00–10:00 AM:	Glass of freshly-squeezed fruit juice: orange, apple, grape, pear, etc. In Chapter 7 you will learn the medicinal value of various juices. Practically any fruit juices can be used, but try to use those which are specifically beneficial for your condition. Juice should be diluted half-and-half with water. *Note!* Avoid commercially bottled, canned or frozen juices.
1:00 PM:	Glass of freshly-made vegetable juice: carrot, celery, tomato, etc., or a mixture of several vegetable juices. Dilute with water. *Or* a cup of vegetable broth.*
4:00 PM:	Cup of herb tea.
7:00 PM:	Glass of freshly-made vegetable or fruit juice, diluted with water.
9:00 PM:	Enema, preferably camomile.

Drink plain lukewarm water when thirsty. The total juice volume during 24 hours should be between 1½ pints and 1½ quarts. Never mix fresh juices with vegetable broth, only with pure water.

This is all.

---

* Wherever they appear throughout the book, asterisks (*) indicate that the recipe or direction cited may be found in Chapter 16.

You may show this book and the instructions in this chapter to your own doctor and ask him to supervise your fasting and examine your condition as your fasting progresses. If you are not able to obtain expert advice, and if you yourself are not sufficiently convinced of the safety and efficiency of this healing measure, I would not advise you to fast longer than one week to ten days at a time.

HOW A FAST IS BROKEN

Note: This is vitally important! *Breaking the fast is the most significant phase of it; the beneficial effects of fasting could be totally undone if the fast is broken incorrectly.*

The main rules of breaking the fast are:

- Do not overeat!
- Chew food extremely well and eat slowly!
- Take several days of gradual transition to the normal diet.

First day, eat one whole apple or other sweet fruit and a little bowl of fresh vegetable soup or puree, unsalted and unspiced, in addition to the usual juice and broth menu.

Second day, you may add to the above some mashed potatoes and a glass of yogurt or homemade soured milk.*

Third day, increase the portions a little and add a small plate of fresh raw vegetable salad, some cooked rice, and a little portion of homemade cottage cheese.*

Fourth day, you can start to eat normally. By normally I mean, of course, that you should continue on the diet recommended in this book. In order to benefit to the greatest possible extent from the therapeutic fasting it is important that after fasting a diet of vital natural foods is maintained. (See Chapter 5.) Such a diet will supply the healing forces of your body with all the vital nutritive elements necessary for the continued repair and healing processes initiated by the body during the fast. However, keep always in mind the first rule of resuming eating after the fast—*do not overeat!* Needless to say, this rule is also the first rule of health.

MORE ADVICE ON FASTING

Should you discontinue with your work and rest or stay in bed during fasting? Not at all! It is advisable to continue with your usual activities, but perhaps avoid too strenuous physical or mental work.

ARCO PUBLISHING COMPANY, INC.
219 Park Avenue South, New York, N.Y. 10003

Daily walks, even long ones for an hour or more, twice a day, are recommended; likewise all suitable exercises. Take a bath two or three times a week, but avoid water too cold or too hot. Dry brushing (see Chapter 11) is recommended morning and evening followed by a shower or wet-towel rub. Plenty of fresh air is extremely important for the healing processes during the fast. For this reason the best time of the year to fast is spring or summer, when you can spend a great deal of time outdoors. Always sleep with an open window.

Fasting will bring about many physiological changes in your body. Increased elimination of toxins through urine, skin and lungs will take place. The body's own healing forces will initiate great repair and health-restoring activity in many ways. These physiological changes may occasionally manifest themselves in certain discomforts such as headache, coated tongue, foul breath, dizziness, or even skin eruptions. These reactions should give no cause for concern. They are common symptoms of fasting and properly understood should not discourage anybody from continuing with the fast.

The first three or four days you will feel hungry, of course. But after that the hunger usually disappears. As a matter of fact, the unbelievable will happen: the longer you fast the less hungry you will feel! When finally the body has completed its repairing and restorative work, it will signal to you by a sudden and definite feeling of hunger that it needs food. This is the physiologically right time to start eating. Of course, in the case of juice fasts even during the first three or four days the patient hardly feels any hunger at all.

Your mental attitude during fasting is of paramount importance. Avoid negative influences. Do not listen to terrified relatives and friends who will warn you that you will pass out any moment. As I said before, nobody has ever died as a result of a few weeks of intentional fasting. Have confidence in what you are doing. Remember, you are not the first to try it—millions of people have done it successfully before you. Even animals fast instinctively when they are sick. But if you do not have complete faith in fasting and are not absolutely convinced of its safety, you should not undertake fasting at all, at least not on your own.

If it makes you feel better do not call this measure a fast. Call it a liquid diet. After all, that is exactly what it is. I know you will be surprised at the results; so will your friends be, especially if you do not tell them you are fasting, but keep it secret. As for myself, I will never stop being amazed at the miraculous prophylactic and healing effects of this, the oldest—and, I dare say, most effective—therapeutic method known to man.

THE EUROPEAN GRAPE CURE

No doubt you have heard of the European Grape Cure. Many books are written on the marvelous benefits and the miraculous healings that have come from living on nothing but grapes for one, two or more weeks. There are many clinics in Europe where you can get a Grape Cure.

There is no doubt that a Grape Cure is an effective treatment in many disorders, from obesity and high blood pressure to arthritis and heart disease. The majority of the biological medical doctors in Europe are, however, of the opinion that the healing effect of the Grape Cure is not as much due to any unusual curative properties of grapes as it is to the modified fasting procedure, which the Grape Cure actually is.

I do not wish to belittle the health-giving value of the grapes. Grapes are, no doubt, a wonderful health food with not only a delicious and satisfying taste but also with a wealth of vitamins, minerals and enzymes. But so are countless other noble fruits and vegetables!

APPLE CURE

A patient I know in Europe cured himself on an Apple Cure. He had very high blood pressure and a heart condition. On the advice of a naturopath, he lived on nothing but ripe sweet apples for several weeks, starting with an apple a day and increasing the apple diet up to two pounds a day. His blood pressure went down and his heart condition improved.

CABBAGE JUICE CURE

I know of a woman who cured herself of stomach ulcers by a Cabbage Juice Cure, and I have heard of an old folk remedy in East Europe where patients with digestive disorders helped themselves to

better health by eating nothing but sauerkraut and drinking the
juice of homemade sauerkraut prepared without salt.

HOW FRUIT AND VEGETABLE JUICE FASTS
WORK FOR YOU

If we analize all these cures we will find that the paramount
feature in all of them is fasting: total, partial or modified—but nevertheless fasting. When you do not consume anything but grapes, or
apples, or carrot juice for prolonged periods of time, your system,
deprived of its "normal" heavy diet of proteins, fats and grains, etc.,
and receiving only easily-assimilated fruits or vegetable juices with
virtually no digestive effort required, will soon institute the process
of autolysis. This is the essential health-restoring activity which the
healing powers of the body institute in order to restore health. By
autolysis, or the process of self-digestion and absorption, the body
breaks down the diseased tissues and burns and excretes the toxic,
morbid matter from the system.

This process of autolysis is to be credited for the miraculous
healing effect of fasting—be it with water, juices, grapes or apples.

People of all ages and in various parts of the world have used
cures with this or that fruit or vegetable without actually realizing
why these cures were so effective. They naturally gave the whole
credit for the cure to the particular fruit, vegetable or drink used.
With the present knowledge of nutrition, biochemistry and the
metabolic and healing processes of the body, it is possible to determine more accurately the exact function of these substances in the
healing processes and give proper credit. The majority of the experienced authorities on fasting agree that although such therapies as
Grape Cure, Apple Cure, Carrot Juice Cure, etc. can be very effective, a more scientific modern fasting on a combination of special
vegetable or fruit juices and mineral-rich, alkaline vegetable broth
gives even better results. For example, in the Buchinger Sanatorium
in Germany, which has the experience of over 70,000 therapeutic
fasts, the intake of juices, broths and herb teas is closely supervised by
doctors in each individual case. Each condition requires a different
regime and a different supply of enzymes, vitamins and minerals for
the maximum curative effect. Special attention is given to mineral
metabolism. Thus, patients with acidosis, or a condition where there
are not enough alkali in the blood, are given alkaline cabbage broth

or other vegetable broths. In cases of mineral deficiency, mineral waters and mineral-rich herb teas are used. In vitamin and enzyme deficiency, raw fruit juices are advised. Various herb teas with particular medicinal properties for different diseases are prescribed individually. This kind of scientific, controlled fasting will, of course, result in faster and more complete recovery.

DO-IT-YOURSELF GRAPE CURE

Since not every one can travel to clinics for fasting, I have described earlier in this chapter how you can undertake fasting on your own in your own home. If you like to try a European Grape Cure, by all means feel free and safe to do it.

Here's how you take a Grape Cure. First, start the treatment with two or three days of fasting, to prepare the system for the change of diet. Then, eat absolutely nothing but grapes for two weeks. The first day, eat only a few for breakfast, a few more for lunch and a couple of ounces for dinner. The second day, eat two or three ounces for each meal. On the third day, increase the portions again. From the fourth and the fifth days on you can eat as many grapes as you desire, within reason, of course, consuming not more than three to four pounds a day. Drink pure water only if and when thirsty.

Here are a few points to remember:

- Eat grapes whole, seeds, skins and all.
- Eat them very slowly, chew well; chew skins thoroughly.
- Seedless varieties are excellent; otherwise chew seeds too. Swallow some, but not all of the seeds.
- Grapes must be 100 percent ripe.
- When completing a Grape Cure, follow the instructions for breaking a juice fast given earlier in this chapter.
- Try to get organically grown grapes from orchards which never use poisonous insecticides or chemical fertilizers. If you use ordinary super-market grapes, wash them carefully to remove traces of insecticides.

3

How to Improve Your Health with Enzymes — Miracle Health Builders

A young Swiss physician was treating an equally young patient who was on the verge of death from starvation because she was unable to digest any kind of food. The disheartened doctor had tried everything, from medication to every imaginable diet, to no avail. The girl could not digest any food whatsoever. Tests in the mornings showed that even the most finely mashed and best cooked food eaten the night before remained wholly undigested in her stomach. The totally emaciated patient was not expected to live more than a few days.

The discouraged young doctor told of his concern for the life of the patient to a friend who was an amateur student of ancient scripts. His friend remembered that in the writings of Pythagoras, an ancient physician of 500 B.C., finely mashed *raw fruits* mixed with *natural honey* and *raw goat's milk* were prescribed in cases of total inability to digest and absorb food. He suggested that the Swiss doctor try this old prescription on his patient.

The doctor was horrified at the suggestion! To fill an impotent digestive system with raw food was against everything he had learned in his medical school, and contrary to the most elementary dietetic rules. The patient was dying, however, and the doctor had nothing else to offer her. There was nothing to lose and everything to gain. He discussed the idea with the patient and she assumed the responsibility for the trial.

The raw food dish, prepared according to Pythagoras' prescription, was given to the patient. The doctor, expecting the worse, kept the patient under close observation. But lo and behold, the tests made the following morning showed that the raw food was completely digested! And the patient felt better! "How could that be?" the shocked doctor asked himself. Exactly the same foods—fruits, milk and honey—in cooked form, given before, were left undigested; and now, the same foods, but fresh and raw, were easily digested and assimilated!

This was a shock for the young physician. He felt that he must find out why the patient could tolerate raw food, but not cooked food. But this was not a time for scientific curiosity—the girl's life was at stake. He continued to feed his patient raw fruits, goat milk and honey. Gradually her digestive organs started to function normally and strength returned to her. Her diet was gradually enlarged to include other foods, mostly in a raw state, until she was completely recovered and regained full health. Her life was saved by a 2,500-year old raw food recipe![1]

DR. MAX BIRCHER-BENNER DISCOVERS "LIFE FORCE"

The young doctor who saved the life of a dying patient with raw foods was a Swiss, Dr. Max Bircher-Benner, who was later to become known in modern text books on nutrition as "a classic in dietetics." He initiated a new school of medical thinking, and during 40 years of practical application and experiments in his clinic in Zurich, proved to his skeptical and conservative colleagues that there are powerful, curative and health-promoting factors in fresh raw foods.

At the time when vitamins and enzymes were yet undiscovered, Dr. Bircher-Benner found that raw foods contained a higher order and quality of nutritive energy, or sun energy, and a life-sustaining and curative power, which were lost in foods subjected to physical and chemical changes such as processing or heating.

This assumption was confirmed 40 years later by several scien-

tific investigations. Nobel Prize-winning physicist Schroedinger, of
Dublin, confirmed that raw foods contain "the life maintaining"
power. Professor Eppinger, of the University of Vienna, showed that
raw food raises the "micro-electric potentials" in living cells.

ENZYMES—THE "LIFE-FORCE" IN RAW FOODS

Dr. Bircher-Benner's discovery, (or I should say "rediscovery,"
since it had been known to ancient physicians) of the healing power
of raw foods was made long before vitamins and enzymes were discovered. Although searching furiously to find out "why," and using
his discovery to help thousands of his patients, Dr. Bircher-Benner
was not able to pinpoint in detail what factors in raw foods were
responsible for their miraculous health-protective and healing properties.

In the last couple of decades nutritional science has leaped for-
ward and advanced at an unprecedented tempo. In 20 years we have
learned more about nutrition than in the previous 20 centuries. Now
we know that the potent "energy" or sun energy, which according to
Bircher-Benner's second principle of thermo-dynamics is lost in foods
subjected to physical and chemical devitalizing processes such as
heating, wilting and industrial processing, comes from natural food's
vital, life-sustaining elements: *enzymes* and *vitamins*.

Enzymes and vitamins are indeed the "Life-Force," the powerful
catalysts which direct and control all life processes in the human
body. Yes, the secret of life itself is in the minute enzyme! Without
enzymes your life would be impossible! Your life depends on adequate nutrition. Your physical energy, your mental capacity, the
proper functioning of your vital organs, the healing and health-restoring processes—all depend on adequate nutrition of vital nutritive
elements. Without enzymes your organism would starve to death,
even if you had plenty to eat, because your body would not be able to
convert foods into energy and into living cells. We talk so much
about vitamins, proteins, and minerals—and they are all essential for
good health and life. But vitamins can work only in the presence of
enzymes. The food you eat must be broken down and changed
chemically into substances which can build the human body. This is
accomplished by the magic work of enzymes.

WHAT ENZYMES ARE AND HOW THEY WORK

You have probably heard references to the human body as a most complicated and intricate piece of machinery. But if you would delve into the deep study of the human enzyme system, you would be astonished and amazed by its ingenious design.

Imagine for a moment an enormous chemical factory where crude raw materials are converted to precious elements through the complicated processes of billions of tiny particles known as enzymes. Your digestive system is such a chemical factory. Follow me on an excursion through it and we trace the process of conversion of crude food into the precious building blocks of your body.

Suppose you eat a simple meal of a cheese sandwich and a glass of milk. As soon as you glance at the menu and decide to order your sandwich—even before it is served to you—your chemical factory starts its work. The complicated machinery of food digestion is *switched on* the moment you make your mental decision to eat a certain food. The enzyme-producing glands located in your stomach and in your mouth are already producing valuable enzymes which will be needed shortly for mastication and swallowing and later for digestion. Enzymes are *catalysts* which bring about chemical changes in food to prepare them for easier digestion and assimilation.

Salivary enzymes

Then the sandwich is served and you take your first bite and drink your milk. As soon as food enters the mouth, several vital enzymes are released by the salivary glands into saliva which will start the digestion of the food even before it enters the stomach. An enzyme called *ptyalin* starts the preliminary work of digestion by attacking immediately the carbohydrates of the bread and breaks them down into *maltose*, the predigested form of starch, or energy-producing sugar.

Stomach enzymes

After it is chewed, the food is swallowed with the help of saliva and enters the stomach. There it is met by various new enzymes which stomach glands were pouring out in anticipation of the food.

Enzyme *rennin* takes care of the milk, causing it to coagulate and changing milk protein, *casein,* into amino acids, a form that your body can use. Rennin also breaks down the minerals of milk and cheese and makes them available for assimilation by the system. These minerals—calcium, phosphorus, magnesium, potassium, etc.— are then transported by the blood stream to become a part of your bones, your teeth, your nerves, and so forth.

Two other enzymes, *pepsin* and *lipase,* help to convert your milk and cheese in the stomach. Pepsin is a foremost digestive enzyme for protein. Lipase works on the fat part of milk and cheese by splitting it into forms which the body uses to nourish its various cells and organs.

But perhaps the most important enzyme in the stomach is *hydrochloric acid.* In addition to its enzymatic action on protein foods and the tough fibrous vegetable cells (in this case on the bran part of the wheat to release wheat proteins, minerals and vitamins) , hydrochloric acid also has other vital functions to perform. By its strong acid nature it destroys bacteria in the stomach, thus acting as a defensive measure against disease-causing bacteria entering your stomach with foods. It also participates in the regulation of the vital acid-alkaline balance in the system. Another important job of hydrochloric acid is to liberate iron from the food and convert it to a form that the body can use.

Intestinal enzymes

After being "worked over" by the powerful stomach enzymes, the partially digested and broken-down food enters the small intestine. Here several new potent enzymes give it a final work-over, and extract and transform the vital nutrients from the food so that they can be assimilated by the blood stream through the intestinal walls and transported to the organs and cells of your body, wherever they are needed.

Bile emulsifies fat from your cheese and milk and prepares it for assimilation. It also assists in the peristaltic processes in the digestive tract. Emulsified fat from the milk and cheese is then subjected to the enzymatic action of *pancreatic lipase,* which breaks fat into fatty acids. It also helps in the assimilation of such fat-soluable vitamins as A, D, and E. After the fats have been changed into useful fatty acids by the action of pancreatic lipase, they are then absorbed by the blood and used in many vital functions of your body: they keep your skin and mucuous membranes in good condition; they are used in building the linings of your nerves and brain tissues; and they play a vital role in healing processes.

Tripsin is another pancreatic enzyme, which continues the digestive work on the proteins of the milk and cheese in your intestines after the preliminary work done by pepsin and rennin in the stomach. And *amylase* gives the final digestive work-over to the starches of your bread.

There are other digestive enzymes in the intestines, such as: *lactase,* which helps to digest the milk sugar, or lactose, in your milk; *streapsin,* which helps in the assimilation of fats from your milk and cheese; *amylopsin,* which helps to assimilate starches from your bread; and many others. Finally, after few hours of elaborate and arduous work by the enzymes—these miracle health builders—your cheese sandwich and glass of milk are transformed to the living tissues in your organs, your skin, your bones, and other parts of your body.

There are over 600 different types of enzymes! And each of them performs a separate vital function. In addition to the all-important digestion and assimilation of food, enzymes are responsible for practically all the vital processes of your body!

Enzymes are present in every cell of your body, and your body is made of billions of cells! Vitamins, minerals, and trace elements are powerless without enzymes. Only as a part of complicated "enzyme systems" can they be triggered into action. Enzymes are responsible for the vital process of autolysis, or self-digestion of diseased and inferior cells and replacement with healthy cells, which occurs during fasting. Without enzymes healing of wounds would be impossible. We know that the proteins in the body are in the so-called *dynamic state.* This means they are being constantly changed from one state to another, being decomposed and resynthesized from the blood plasma amino acid. This process is accomplished by enzymes.

Without enzymes your body cannot convert food into energy and into the living cells of the body. Enzymes transform proteins, carbohydrates, fats, vitamins and other nutrients into your muscles, bones, hair, skin, organs, glands, hormones, blood, etc.

If to all this you add the fact that enzymes protect you against inflammations, promote healing, dissolve clots and tumors, "erase" scars, counteract the adverse effects of drugs, aid in formation of urea and passing it off in urine, aid in blood coagulation, promote oxygenation of blood and tissues, are involved in your sexual libido, are directly responsible for your general state of health—then you realize the miraculous power of these tiny substances!

Enzymes are responsible for the normal healthy function of all your bodily processes, for your mental and physical health. They have the power to rejuvenate your entire being, or, conversely, to cause premature aging and death.

WHERE DO ENZYMES COME FROM?

Your body can manufacture many enzymes from the food you eat, water you drink and air you breathe. Enzymes are also present in all natural foods in their *raw* state. When you eat raw foods, you are supplying your digestive system with the enzymes necessary for the effective digestion and assimilation of the nutrients from these foods. Note that enzymes must be replenished all the time. After enzymes complete their particular work, they are destroyed and the body has to manufacture new enzymes.

There are *endogenous enzymes,* or those found within the body, and *exogenous enzymes,* which are found in raw foods. Both have similar properties, and the more enzymes supplied with the foods you eat, the more easily and effectively can your body conduct its vital processes. In a condition of ill health, especially when digestive organs are diseased and unable to digest foods properly, the enzymes in raw foods are able to duplicate the functions of endogenous enzymes and assist in digestion and assimilation of the nutrients from the food in which they appear.

HOW ENZYMES ARE DESTROYED

Enzymes are present only in natural, unprocessed foods. Heating, cooking, canning, pasteurization, and processing destroy enzymes. Temperatures over 122° F are lethal to enzymes. This means that when you cook your fruits, vegetables or other foods, all enzymes are permanently destroyed.

Therefore, if you want to benefit from the powerful effect of enzymes on your health, you have to eat your foods in their natural, raw state. You may say that you can't eat all foods raw, they would be unpalatable. Unpalatable, yes! I am glad you brought it up! Perhaps this is the only really dependable guiding rule as to which foods were intended by the Creator to be eaten by humans. All fruits, vegetables, nuts, seeds, honey, etc. are actually more delicious and palatable raw than cooked. And, of course, all raw foods are much easier to digest than cooked foods—provided your digestive system is not totally degenerated and diseased by the prolonged use of cooked and devitalized foods.

In order to give your digestive system time to rebuild itself and adjust to the new diet, it would be best to make a gradual transition from predominantly cooked and processed foods to raw foods. Start by adding more and more raw foods to your menu, and gradually arrive at the point where at least two-thirds of all your food is in a raw state. This is not difficult to achieve, since all fruits, vegetables, berries, milk and nuts, and most grains and seeds can be eaten raw. (The best way to eat grains is to sprout them—see Chapter 16 for instructions.)

Wild animals, who in their wild state eat only raw natural foods, do not become sick. When the same animals are kept in zoos and fed cooked food, they suddenly develop the same diseases which civilized man suffers from: cancer, tuberculosis, rheumatic diseases, etc. Very often the captive animals in zoos become sterile. Zoos today are learning to apply this knowledge by feeding animals *raw* foods and keeping them healthy.

There is no doubt that the day man learned how to cook his food he brought upon himself disease and premature death. "Primitive" man lived on raw fruits, nuts, berries, honey, and raw milk. He used ancient methods of preserving by fermentation. The word *enzyme* comes from the Greek *enzymos,* which means *ferment* or *leaven.* Man used enzymes, or ferments, to make sour milk and cheese. He fermented bread and made it rise with the help of enzymes. He preserved vegetables by the enzymatic process of "pickling" them, or making sauerkraut, sour pickles, etc. All these foods are storehouses of enzymes. Man knew no disease and lived to a great age, as we are told in mythology and in the Bible. Even today, Eskimos and many tribes of Africa and Central America who eat practically all their food raw, do not suffer from the diseases of civilized man, who largely exists on cooked food. Cooking destroys not only enzymes, but also vitamins, and changes proteins and fats to a form more difficult to digest.

Now you can see why the young lady I was telling you about in the beginning of this chapter, who was dying from the inability of her organs to digest food, was saved by the raw food diet. The enzymatic system of this girl was paralyzed and out of order. Her stomach glands were not producing the enzymes necessary for the digestion of food. The foods her doctor was giving her were all well-cooked and *totally void of enzymes*. Naturally they stayed in her stomach undigested. When she received a dish of raw fruits, raw goat milk, and raw honey, foods containing all the enzymes necessary for their own digestion, these foods were, in fact, capable of digesting themselves! Both honey and raw fruits require virtually no digestion. Honey and fruit juices are absorbed directly to the blood stream "without digestion" due to their predigested form. And goat milk is now known to be a highly concentrated source of enzymes!

A 10-POINT PROGRAM
TO GET ENOUGH ENZYMES
FOR HEALTHFUL LIVING

Here is a 10-point program which will assure you a generous supply of enzymes—the miracle health builders:

1. Eat as much raw food as possible. At least 50 percent, but still better two-thirds of your diet should be raw. This is not nearly as difficult to achieve as it may seem. Never cook fruits and vegetables. Why destroy these excellent foods when they not only taste better raw but also are more easily digested in a raw form? Learn to prepare delicious fresh vegetable and fruit salads. Bircher-Benner Müesli* and Fruit Salad à la Airola* are powerful storehouses of enzymes.

2. Eat foods as soon as possible after they have been harvested. Keep raw foods chilled all of the time. Storage and wilting destroy some of the enzymes.

3. In winter, or when raw fruits and vegetables are scarce, use frozen foods. Freezing does not destroy enzymes, only inactivates them. However, they disappear rapidly when frozen food is thawed—eat it immediately!

4. If you must cook some of the vegetables, cook them as fast and as little as possible. Chinese cooking, which leaves vegetables still crisp and half raw, preserves part of the enzymes.

5. Chew all your foods well, especially carbohydrate foods: fruits, vegetables, seeds and grains. Enzymatic action on foods starts in your mouth!

---

* Wherever they appear throughout the book, asterisks (*) indicate that recipes or directions cited are to be found in Chapter 16.

6. Use unpasteurized raw milk and natural cheese only. Pasteurization and cheese-processing destroy enzymes. Goat milk is particularly rich in enzymes. Raw milk is available at better health food stores.

7. Use as many as possible of the "fermented" enzyme-foods: homemade sauerkraut,* homemade soured milk,* homemade yogurt,* homemade kefir,* homemade cottage cheese,* and homemade sour pickles.* These foods are potent sources of beneficial enzymes and are practically predigested foods which require very little digestion in the stomach. They are also extremely beneficial for the healthy condition of the bacterial flora in the digestive tract.

8. Raw grains, especially wheat, and seeds are rich sources of enzymes. Since baking requires high temperatures, bread is void of enzymes. Use grains raw. There are many ways to do it. Sprouted wheat* or other sprouted grains are delicious foods and are literally loaded with enzymes. Bircher-Benner Müesli,* which contains raw oats, is a powerful source of enzymes.

9. Buy a juice extractor and make your own enzyme-loaded drinks: fresh raw fruit and vegetable juices. Carrots, cabbage, celery, tomatoes, apples, pineapples, pears, and grapes are especially appropriate for juicing. Use separately or mix them to suit your taste. But never mix raw vegetables and raw fruits together, in juicing or eating. Drink juices between meals, or before meals, but not after. Drink juices immediately after they have been prepared.

10. Supplement your diet with the following special foods rich in exogenous enzymes:

- Brewer's yeast—rich in enzymes, B-vitamins, and complete proteins.
- Honey, raw, unprocessed, unheated—rich in enzymes, vitamins, and pollen.
- Papaya—an excellent source of papain, enzyme needed for protein digestion. Papaya juice is sold in health food stores.
- Rose hips—a rich source of vitamins C and P, and enzymes.
- Kelp—rich in minerals, iodine, vitamins and enzymes.

All these special food supplements are, in addition to enzymes, extremely rich in vitamins and minerals, which are coenzymes; that is, they help the enzymes in their work.

4

Water — Nature's Wonder Healer

Once upon a time (until about 25–30 years ago) the United States had many well-known and well-frequented spas. Dr. Kellog's Battle Creek Spa was one of the most familiar ones. Many others were active in Florida, near Chicago and on the West Coast. Most of them were operated by Europeans who migrated from Western Europe and brought with them the experience of similar watering places in the old country. Millions of people visited these spas, took baths or "cures," and relieved themselves of aches and pains, of arthritis and high blood pressure, of depression and eczema.

But with the advent of the chemical takeover of medicine these spas have now almost completely disappeared from the American scene. An average American wouldn't think of "tampering" with his health by going to a water cure spa or taking a mineral bath—any more than he would try to improve his health by eating organically grown foods. These things are strictly for the "health nuts"!

WATER CURE SPAS IN EUROPE

In Europe millions of people each year go to health spas, *"Bads,"* or water resorts and take a water cure. Over 3,000,000 people in West Germany alone visit *Bads* each year.

The water cure is an old tradition in Europe. Cities have been built around mineral-rich springs. You have only to take a quick look at the German map to notice hundreds of towns and cities with the prefix *"Bad"* (spa) to its name, like Bad Neuenhahr, Bad Pyrmont, Bad Homburg, or with a suffix like Wiesbaden or plain Baden-Baden. Only when spring waters are medically recognized as being of therapeutic value may the town add the prefix *Bad* to its name. Some of these are big cities, like Wiesbaden, with a population of 260,000; some are just small villages with a few hotels for the water cure guests.

People travel to these spas on their own or on the recommendation of their doctors. Most *Bads* have several clinics and sanatoriums where medical doctors give an examination and advise on drinking waters from certain springs and/or using various other water cure facilities: baths, packs, swimming, steam inhaling, etc. The pleasant atmosphere of a typical beautiful resort town with many parks and lakes for walks and recreation, adds to the overall curative and health-restoring atmosphere.

BAD PYRMONT

I have visited many *Bads* in Germany. One of the most typical and the most delightful places I have seen is Bad Pyrmont, near Hanover, in the Lower Saxon State.

The picturesque town of Bad Pyrmont is beautifully located in the valley between forest-clad hills. The spa is state-owned and operated, but the town has many private clinics and sanatoriums. During the high season for cures, about 80 percent of the town's population are patients and guests.

Here are some excerpts from the information brochure published by the state government for the benefit of those who seek the water cure at Bad Pyrmont:

"Be healthy and keep fit! Visit Bad Pyrmont for disorders of the heart and blood, women's complaints and rheumatism."

"A typical family goes to Bad Pyrmont in search of health and recuperation and to experience its wonderful curative powers." —

"New balneological† discoveries are combined with the experience of centuries."

"Bad Pyrmont is ideal for all—the sick and the healthy who know that prevention is better than cure, the young and the old."

"Bay Pyrmont Spa facilities are recommended for the treatment of the following diseases:

"Diseases of the heart and circulation; cardiac insufficiency, cardiac infarct, coronary thrombosis, disorders in blood pressure, peripheral circulation disorders, nervous disorders of the heart and circulation. Diseases of the blood-forming organs. All types of anemia. Rheumatic diseases of the bones, joints and muscles. Women's complaints: inflammation of female abdominal organs, periodic and other hormone disorders. Eczema. Allergies. Conditions of exhaustion. Children's diseases. Diseases of old age and senility."

Keep in mind that this is not a "quack"-operated joint trying to cheat people of their money by offering a bogus water cure for all these serious diseases, *but a state-operated establishment that has been approved by the State Medical Association!*

The spa offers the following treatments:

"Carbonic acid chalybeate springs for baths and drinking cures. Saline and brine springs for saline baths, drinking and inhalation cures. Carbonic acid gas from the springs for baths. Chalybeate peat for baths (deep and partial immersion) and packs. Mixed baths.

"Supplementary treatments; inhalation cures in single cabins and public inhalatorium. Oral douches for pyorrhea. Massage. Undercurrent massage and douches. Colonic irrigation. Arm baths (Hauffe) . Alternate hot-and-cold foot baths. Hydrotherapy. Vaginal douches. Terrain cures. Special diets. Rest cures. Gymnastics (Medau method) . Sun and air baths."

DO MINERAL WATERS "WORK"?

If they didn't, it would be unlikely that over three million people in West Germany alone would visit spas every year, year after year.

I have talked to doctors in Bad Pyrmont and their reaction to my question was something like this:

---

† Balneology—medical science of curing and preventing sickness by bathing.

The modern inquiry into balneology and the medicinal value of mineral waters is recent and as yet incomplete. But what is already known indicates that mineral waters do indeed have curative powers. And they should, inasmuch as disordered mineral metabolism and biochemical derangement are at the root of many diseases. But what is even more important is the fact that these waters here in Bad Pyrmont have been used for healing purposes for almost two thousand years; and millions of sick people have been benefited by them—patients and doctors see examples of it every day!

I have asked some patients for the reasons for coming to Bad Pyrmont, and here are a few of the answers I received:

"I have high blood pressure," said a stout, executive-looking gentleman. "Medication does not help me at all. Also, I have a weight problem. So my doctors advised me to come here. I come each summer and take the water cure for six weeks. In that time my blood pressure usually goes down to normal and I lose some weight. By the next spring my blood pressure probably will go up again, so I'll make another visit here. These mineral waters keep me alive!"

"I have been suffering from arthritis for three years," said a young-looking blonde lady of approximately 30. "I am staying at the sanatorium here and taking a cure under my doctor's supervision. I have been fasting three weeks and drinking mineral waters. I have also taken many different kinds of baths and water treatments. My arthritis is almost gone. All the pain disappeared after the first week here. I hardly could bend my knees before; now I walk all day long without any discomfort."

I stopped a little girl of about seven, who was on the way to the bath appointment with her mother. "My girl had a disfiguring eczema for several months. Our doctor didn't know the cause of it and was unable to help her with drugs, so he sent us here. Now she has been taking baths, packs, and drinking cures for six weeks and her eczema is almost gone. Only a very few small spots are left on her elbows."

On a bench in the beautiful spa park I talked to a group of elderly people, the patients at the state-operated rehabilitation clinic for heart diseases. They all had long records of cardiac insufficiency, circulatory problems and blood pressure disorders. They were sent there by their medical insurance government each year to improve their health and particularly to improve their heart condition. They all assured me that they felt "so much better" after staying one month at their clinic and taking all the recommended water cures.

SANATORIUM DR. BUCHINGER

One of the most famous sanatoriums in Bad Pyrmont is a huge, ultra-modern clinic directed by Dr. Otto H. F. Buchinger. The clinic is equipped according to the latest principles of diagnostic practice and staffed with experienced medical, nursing, and technical staffs.

Although the Buchinger Sanatorium is internationally known for its medicinal fasts, the hydrotherapeutic treatments occupy a central place in his clinic: colonic irrigation, mud packs, underwater massage, "mesenchymal massage," oxygen baths, carbon dioxide mixture baths, herb tea scrub baths, sauna, and all the water applications according to the late Pastor Kneipp.

Dr. Buchinger showed me his spotlessly clean, beautiful and luxurious clinic and talked at length about his experience with fasting: "Together with my father, also a medical doctor, I have supervised somewhere between 70 and 80 thousand fasts. In my experience, the best results with fasting can be obtained with mineral water and juices. The establishing of proper mineral balance in the blood and tissues is of utmost importance for the maximum result in therapeutic fasting. The mineral-rich waters here, with low sodium content, and the vegetable juices and teas, particularly cabbage juice and peppermint tea, help us to achieve remarkable results in the treatment of almost all acute or chronic diseases: heart and circulatory diseases, rheumatic diseases, high blood pressure, chronic skin disorders, nervous disorders, etc."

MEDICAL SCIENCE DISCOVERS
THE VALUE OF WATER SPAS

In an article called "Effect of a French Mineral Water on Serum Cholesterol,"[1] Drs. Korenyi, Harkavy and Whittier reported on the experiments they conducted with 34 patients with high cholestrol levels at the Creedmoor State Hospital in New York. These patients, whose serum cholesterol levels were above 240 mg. percent, did not receive any other type of treatment known to have any effect on serum cholesterol, except 30½ fluid ounces of mineral water daily in three divided doses. The treatment continued for 30 days.

At the end of two weeks the average decrease of serum cholesterol was 9.9 mg. percent. At the conclusion of the study, the average decrease was 23.8 mg. percent.

A Hungarian doctor, O. Schulhof, M.D., made a study of the spa therapies and reported that "beside the psychological effects produced by the changed environment, and the complex effect of combined drug, electro- and mechano-therapeutic treatments, we still attribute importance to the specific effect of the mineral water." Dr. Schulhof said that it has been demonstrated that mineral water is actually absorbed through the skin. Mineral waters have been shown to have a beneficial effect on the connective tissues as well as on the immunological and healing powers of the body.

The doctors in Hungary have discovered that patients taking cortisone can do as well without it after taking the spa treatment. "By spa hospital treatment it is often possible for patients who have taken corticosteroids for years to do without them; one might say that by means of spa therapy we can carry out 'corticosteroid withdrawal' treatment."[2]

In Russia, there are several research centers where balneology, the medical science of curing and preventing sickness by the use of water, is studied. Russia has hundreds of government-operated spas and bathing clinics. Over six million people go to these spas and bathing resorts each year and take "the cure." Russian scientists believe that the best way to prevent disease is to stimulate the body's own defensive and resistant forces. "Among these stimulating agencies the first place belongs to spa treatment and rest," said the Russian Academy of Sciences, Soviet's highest scientific institution.

People have been using mineral springs and various kinds of water baths for ages, long before civilization. In the Caucasus Mountains you can see ancient bathing places where cave dwellers carried their sick to bathe in natural hot springs. Mexican Indians used natural hot springs and mineral waters for the healing of the sick long before the white man stepped on this continent. Man throughout his history has instinctively appreciated the invigorating and rejuvenating effect of hot and cold baths in springs, rivers, lakes, and oceans.

PRIESSNITZ, WATER CURE PIONEER

An Austrian layman, Vincenz Priessnitz, 1799–1851, may be regarded as the first to bring the water cure to the attention of the European medical doctors and to give it a scientific respectability. His water treatments were aimed at stimulating and encouraging sluggish vital organs to better eliminating activity. He used various cold water applications to accomplish this: total immersion; partial baths for feet, arms, head or any other affected part; packs with wet sheets; cold compresses; cold douches; etc. In 1826, Priessnitz built the original water cure establishment at Grafenberg, where many doctors from around the world came to study his methods. Soon water cure establishments sprang up all over the world.

FATHER KNEIPP

Another and perhaps better known pioneer of water cure methods was Father Kneipp, of Woerishofen, Bavaria. He may be better known for another of his treatments: walking barefoot in dewy grass. Father Kneipp achieved great fame and a large following by the successful application of his water cures in many difficult cases. Even today, thousands of people from all over the world travel to Woerishofen to take Father Kneipp's famous water cures.

"Water contains great healing power," said Father Kneipp. According to his theory, fresh, cool, "living" water improves circulation in the feet, legs and internal organs and speeds the healing processes. Patients at Father Kneipp's clinic use natural sun-drenched waters of creeks and streams to stimulate their circulation.

THE VALUE OF SUN-DRENCHED "LIVING" WATER

There is a growing conviction among people and practitioners that "living," sun-drenched water from fast-flowing streams and lakes, replenished by rainfall and irradiated by sunlight, has a special curative property—in both internal and external use.

There are many theories as to why *living* water is better for health and healing. One is that sunlight has an enriching effect on

water, which absorbs solar energy. This energy influences the growth
and reproduction of beneficial microorganisms which exercise a
destructive influence on disease-causing organisms that pollute water.
Another theory for the curative power of living water is that rain
water and water from open springs, pools and rivers is a potent
source of oxygen and beneficial microorganisms from the air in
addition to the vital solar energy. When man began drinking under-
ground water he lost some of his hereditary resistance to disease,
which is still possessed by wild animals who drink living water.[3]

The great ancient physicians Hippocrates and Galen believed in
the healing power of living water. The Greeks cured themselves by
drinking water from the healing fountains in the temples, where
running water was given the maximum of aeration and exposure to
sunlight.

SITZ BATH

In European clinics and *kurorts* sitz baths have a specially preferred position. There are three forms of sitz baths: warm, cold, and
alternate hot and cold sitz baths.

The hot sitz bath is beneficial for relieving pain and inflammation in the reproductive organs and other organs of the pelvic region.
The water should be as hot as can be borne comfortably and the
duration of the bath from 10 to 15 minutes.

The cold sitz bath has a stimulating and invigorating effect on
the reproductive organs and the spine. It is popularly called a "youth
bath," because it has a rejuvenating effect as the result of increasing
blood circulation to the vital centers. Many men have found that
cold sitz baths have banished their "bedroom fatigue" and increased
their libido. The temperature of the water should be 50–65 degrees
and the duration of the bath from three to five minutes. After the
bath rub yourself dry and warm with a coarse bath towel.

The alternate hot and cold sitz bath is best for patients with
lowered vitality. This bath requires two tubs: one containing hot
and the other cold water. The patient first sits in the hot water for 10
to 15 minutes, then changes to the cold for half a minute. Make three
to four changes, always finishing with the cold water.

Here's how you can take a do-it-yourself sitz bath in your own
home without a special tub:

Fill your bathtub with water about eight inches high, or a little less than half-full. Sit in the tub with your knees drawn up so that only the "sitz" and the feet are covered by the water. For patients in a weak condition, it is advisable to place their feet in a small tub or pan filled with warm water.

A sitz bath can be taken two or three times a week.

COLD SHOWER

The invigorating, rejuvenating and health-restoring power of hot and cold water is well established—both by tradition and the experiences of thousands of years of actual application, and by the studies of modern science. In Chapter 8 I will tell you of the magic power of the overheating baths for healing purposes. In this chapter so far I have shown you several ways of using cold water for improving or restoring your health. One of the simplest and easiest forms of homemade water cure treatment is an ordinary shower.

Cold shower treatment has a special tonic-like magic of exerting an exceedingly beneficial effect on the entire system. Here's what a simple good old cold shower can do for you:

- It will stimulate circulation and increase muscle tone and nerve force.
- It will stimulate the glandular system, especially the adrenal glands, to increased hormone production.
- It will speed metabolism and improve digestion.
- It has a powerful influence on the central nervous system, the brain, and all the vital organs of the body.
- It will build up your resistance against colds and infections.
- It will help to prevent premature aging and keep you younger longer.

As you see, it is a real life-elixir! And it's free and so easy to take!

In Swedish biological clinics the cold shower is used extensively, especially in treatment of rheumatic diseases.

A cold shower is a real beauty bath, too. The cold water on the upturned face is one of the best beauty treatments known. It tightens the skin, prevents wrinkles and promotes a healthy, radiant complexion. Even if you take a warm bath or shower, always finish with a cold shower, at least on the face.

It has been shown that a cold shower actually increases the blood count. Some doctors also claim that a cold shower is mildly electronic in action and increases the intake of oxygen to a remarkable degree. And, as you know, oxygen is life itself. The more oxygen in your blood and your cells, the better your health.

So, by all means, treat yourself to a cold shower—this simplest and cheapest water cure method—each morning and evening!

Dr. Henry Lindlahr summed the value of a water cure, based on his own experience, in these words: "There is no such thing as a 'cure-all'—any remedy or panacea for all ailments—*but if there were* such a thing, it would be cold water, properly applied."

SALT WATER BATH

Perhaps of all natural living waters salt sea water has the greatest curative power.

We all have experienced the invigorating effect of a few days or weeks by the seashore. The reasons are obvious: It has been shown that minerals are absorbed through the skin and also through the inhaled mineral-rich air by the seashore.

Sea water is extremely rich in beneficial minerals. One to two teaspoons a day can be used internally as a mineral supplement. Make every effort to spend your holiday by the sea. In addition to providing the usual benefits of cold water bathing, salt water and salt air will recharge your system with health-restoring and rejuvenating minerals.

HOMEMADE SALT WATER BATH

If you are not fortunate enough to live near the ocean, here is an easy do-it-yourself salt water bath which you can enjoy right in your own bathtub.

Three or four pounds of sea salt is dissolved in a tub half-full of cool water. Enjoy salt water swimming by rubbing yourself briskly, then drying yourself warm with coarse towels. If sea salt is not available (health food stores are the most likely places to find it), the following ingredients can be substituted for it:

3½ lb. common salt
½ lb. magnesium chloride
½ lb. Epsom salts

SALT WATER SAND PACKS

I have told about mud pack cures used in European biological clinics. But in Mexico I learned a wonderful way to make a do-it-yourself sand pack cure by the seashore. On my favorite beach in San Blas, Nayarit, I have on several occasions observed Indians from nearby mountains coming down to the ocean and taking these packs. This is how they do it:

They dig a hole in the sand sufficiently deep for a man to lie down flat in it. The hole should be close enough to the water so that the bottom of the hole will be moist from the seeping sea water. The patient lies down in the hole and is completely covered by the dry hot sand, leaving only the face uncovered. Then the others bring a pail of sea water and pour it over the sand. The patient stays in the hole for about 15 minutes to half an hour.

I have asked several Indians why they take these packs. Their answer was always enthusiastic: These sand packs have a wonderful healing effect on most diseases, but especially on abdominal disorders, nervous conditions and blood diseases. They have told me of many dramatic cases of miraculous cures accomplished by these packs. There is no doubt that the combination of the osmotic absorption of minerals from the sea water and the therapeutic effect of cold water and hot sand packs has a powerful healing effect. Try a salt water sand pack next time you are on the beach!

By the way, these same Indians always take several bottles of sea water with them to the mountains. They told me that they drink it when they feel "out of sorts."

PSAMOTOTHERAPY

On Gran Canaria, Canary Islands, I have visited the Heliotherapeutic Center where they give hot sand treatments. There are only two heliotherapeutic treatment establishments in the world: one in Italy and this one on the marvelous sunny beach of Maspalomas, Gran Canaria, where there is clear, hot sunny weather 365 days of the year! An ideal place for psamototherapy, or sand treatment. The treatments are exceptionally beneficial for all forms of rheumatic diseases and arthritis. Patients are put in a hole dug in the sand hill and covered by hot sand. The sand is previously sprayed with sea water and seaweed extract. Again, the treatment consists of a combination of minerals from sea water and heat.

SULPHUR BATH

Sulphur baths are used in the treatment of skin disorders, nervous conditions, neuritis and rheumatic diseases. Drug stores carry ready-made fluid preparations for sulphur baths; use accordingly to directions. If you can't obtain a ready-made preparation, use the following formula: take two ounces of *potassium sulphide* and dissolve in 15 gallons of water, which is a little over one-half tub full.

SUMMARY:
HOW TO USE WATER—NATURE'S WONDER HEALER— TO PREVENT AND CURE DISEASE

1. The modern science of balneology has confirmed the experience of centuries that natural mineral waters do indeed possess curative properties. Millions of Europeans visit thousands of water cure spas on the recommendation of their doctors and testify that the water cure indeed "works."

2. Although most spas have disappeared from the American scene, there are still a few left, such as Saratoga Spa in New York and a few in Florida. If you are one of those "who have tried everything and nothing has helped," perhaps a visit to a mineral water spa will help you. Or why not spend a few weeks at some of the famous Bads in Europe on your next holiday trip there? You will find them in abundance in every European country, but particularly in Germany.

3. Do-it-yourself sitz baths, described in this chapter, are easy to take and the benefits from them could be a real surprise to you. Give them a try. Many tired men have sitz baths to thank for their renewed vigor.

4. Father Kneipp's famous "living" water cures are as easy as they are delightful, especially barefoot walking in the dewy grass. Millions of enthusiastic followers of his teachings can't all be wrong. Try it!

5. Try a homemade salt water bath and a sulphur bath. They are backed by a long record of successful application. Remember: it has been proved that minerals are absorbed through the skin.

6. Use every opportunity to spend some time by the seashore. Salt sea water and salt-filled air are stimulating and rejuvenating elixirs. Take one or two teaspoons of pure sea water each day with your meals. Sea water is the best mineral supplement you can think of.

7. Finally, if none of the above "turns you on," the least you can do is to take cold showers in your own bath room each morning and evening. Don't be deceived by the simplicity of this water cure— it has a magic revitalizing and rejuvenating effect on all the vital organs and on the entire system.

Here is an ideal combination of exercise, dry brush massage, and cold showers for each morning and evening:

a) Do your usual exercises, isometric or conventional, until you feel all warmed up.

b) Brush your whole body with a stiff-bristled brush. (See Chapter 11 for instructions.)

c) Take an alternate warm and cold shower, finishing with water as cold as you can stand.

d) Rub yourself dry and warm with a coarse towel.

This simple routine will build up your resistance to colds and infections, save you money on doctors' bills, stimulate the functions of all your vital organs and glands, improve your spirits and disposition, and help to prevent premature aging—in short it will keep you **younger longer!**

5

How You Can Help Regain Health and Freedom from Disease Through the European Waerland Health System

In contrast to most health systems which are limited in scope and which one-sidedly stress certain health-promoting factors—diet, exercise, yoga, baths, etc., (all important and vital factors, of course)—the Waerland system is a complete health system which takes all the factors related to man's physical and emotional health into consideration. It is a health system based on an idea of "wholeness," which embraces all health factors, both of the mind and the body.

Waerland himself has expressed his philosophy in a nutshell in the following sentence:

We do not deal with disease—only with mistakes in our way of living; eliminate the mistakes and the diseases will disappear of their own accord.

Waerland's advice to the members of the healing professions was not to cure a disease, but to cure a sick body. And the sick body can be cured not by seeking to get rid of the symptoms by means of drugs, but by correcting man's faulty living habits and restoring his original biological rhythm of working and living. Thus the Waerland health system incorporates the following health-promoting factors:

- Natural, health-giving foods.
- Plenty of fresh air day and night, and sufficient exposure to sun.
- Sufficient physical work and exercise.
- A clean body through baths and dry brushing.
- Efficient bowel elimination through a lacto-vegetarian diet and plenty of raw vegetables and fruits.
- Positive mental attitude based on belief in man's divinely designed calling as a human being.

Those who are in good health will be able to prevent ill health and disease by following this total health program. To those who are suffering ill health, the application of these health-restoring factors will bring them back into harmony with their natural environment, "eliminate the mistakes in their way of living" and restore and build their health.

"Man's health is his birthright," says Are Waerland. Man brought disease upon himself by disobeying the God-given laws of nature. Eliminate the mistakes in your way of living and attune yourself with the laws of health and all diseases will disappear.

WAERLAND DIET-SYSTEM IN A NUTSHELL[1]

Morning

On awaking in the morning take one to one and a half cups of the Waerland drink, "Excelsior."* This is a very alkaline drink composed of vegetable broth plus flaxseed and wheat bran. It neutralizes over-acidity, helps in elimination of harmful metabolic toxins, and stimulates peristaltic bowel movements, thus helping to relieve constipation. "Excelsior" is prepared in the evening and stored in the refrigerator. Warm it up in the morning to body temperature and drink it all, seeds and bran, without chewing.

Morning routine

First, *head massage*. Using circular movements with your finger tips, massage firmly from the neck and the temples to the crown of

---

* Wherever they appear, asterisks (*) indicate that the recipe or direction cited may be found in Chapter 16.

the head. This stimulates hair growth and improves mental activity by bringing more blood to your head.

Next, a *cold shower* or cold rub-down with a sponge; finish with a vigorous drying with a rough towel.

After shower, a *dry-brush massage*. Use a stiff, bristle brush (not nylon) and brush vigorously all over the body from top to toe. (See Chapter 11.)

Morning *exercises* are next. These could be any of your own favorite gymnastics, or a short, brisk morning walk.

Breakfast

Waerland does not advocate a large breakfast. The morning hours, until 11 or 12 o'clock, constitute a period of elimination, when the bloodstream is heavily charged with the waste products of metabolism and the organs are doing their job of eliminating impurities and toxins from the system. A large breakfast may disrupt this process and interrupt elimination. Therefore it is essential to have a breakfast which requires the minimum of digestive effort and, at the same time, has a cleansing effect on the digestive system.

Homemade soured milk,* yogurt,* or buttermilk in combination with fresh juicy fruits, such as apples, pears, grapefruit, oranges, bananas, grapes, or fresh berries, is an ideal breakfast.

If fruits are not available, soured milk could be eaten with finely-cut onions stirred into it and then topped with powdered dried nettles, alfalfa, or rose hip powder, and wheat bran, wheat germ, and milk sugar (lactose). Unsprayed and unsulphured dried fruits, such as figs, currants, raisins, prunes, apricots, etc., are also excellent in combination with soured milk. Wash them well and soak in cold water overnight.

Between-meal snacks and drinks

No between-meal snacks are recommended with the exception of fresh fruit.

Herb teas are very beneficial between meals. Use any of the teas available at health food stores, or make your own from unsprayed leaves of apples, raspberries, black currants, birch, strawberries, etc. Rose hip tea* is especially recommended for its delicious flavor, aroma and large amount of natural Vitamin C. Use honey to sweeten your tea.

Lunch

A bowl of Five-Grain Kruska,* or Uncooked Quick Kruska.*
Kruska can be eaten with sweet, unpasteurized milk and stewed fruits, or dried fruits soaked overnight. Homemade applesauce* is an ideal addition to Kruska.

Kruska is a highly nutritious and heavy meal in itself. If desired, however, it could be supplemented with wholemeal bread* and butter, and with freshly sliced onions and a mild cheese, preferably homemade cottage cheese.*

There are various ways to prepare Kruska and each individual must experiment to determine the type of Kruska which is best adapted to his needs.

Dinner

The standard Waerland dinner consists of a large bowl of fresh vegetable salad, the emphasis being on green leafy vegetables. The foundation of this alkaline vegetable meal is a large portion of unpeeled potatoes, either baked in the oven or boiled. Three other standard ingredients are grated raw carrots, red beets and onions. Cabbage, curly kale, chives, raddish, lettuce, dill, parsley and garlic are excellent additions to the salad. Use any available fresh vegetables.

In addition to the potatoes and salad, one could eat one or two slices of sour-dough rye bread* with butter and freshly-cut slices of onions and mild cheese, or cottage cheese. Sour milk or yogurt combine excellently with this vegetable meal, but sweet milk is not allowed. Enzymes and acidophilus bacteria of sour milk have been shown to assist in the digestion and assimilation of raw vegetables.

Note: no drinks of any kind; no vinegar, lemon juice, sugar, raisins, or fresh fruits should be used with this raw vegetable meal. Cooked fruits can be used for dessert, if desired. An exception is made for persons with hydrochloric acid deficiency; in such cases it is permissible to use a little freshly squeezed lemon juice as a dressing for salads. Also, a little cranberry sauce could be used by such persons as a stimulus to the hydrochloric acid glands.

Don'ts of Waerland diet-system

- No salt, vinegar, pepper, mustard, or other sharp spices or condiments.

- No coffee, tea, tobacco, or alcohol.
- No white sugar or anything made with it; sweets, candies, chocolate, cakes, ice cream, cookies and such.
- No white bread or anything made with white flour.
- No canned, processed, refined or adulterated foods.
- No meat, fish or eggs.

Change-over period

During a change-over period from the "ordinary" diet to the Waerland system, it is important, especially for sick persons, to cleanse the body of accumulated toxins, impurities and residues of sluggish metabolism. Enemas, fasting and lots of exercise in fresh air are helpful for this purpose. The description of fasting in Chapter 2 of this book can be used as a guide in this respect.

WHY AND HOW TO TAKE AN ENEMA

Practically all conditions which lead to chronic diseases are the result of accumulated impurities (toxins) in the body. Constipation is one of the most common ailments of civilized man. As a consequence of long-standing constipation, the digestive tract, particularly in the lower bowels and colon, becomes slack and stagnant, with hardened residues clinging to the walls of the colon and filling its many pockets and folds. Also, excrements tend to collect and remain too long in the sigmoid (the S-looking curve just above the rectum). This results in putrefaction and gas, forming a source of slow poisoning of the whole body.

Therefore, it is essential that the digestive and eliminative system is restored to a normal condition if positive results of the change-over to the Waerland diet are to be expected. Enemas can do much to restore effective elimination.

To take an enema, you must have an enema can with a rubber hose and a nozzle; it can be obtained at any drug store. First, take one pint of luke warm water (about 99° F) with a few drops of lemon juice. The best position for taking an enema is on your knees, head down to the floor, with a can standing or hanging two to three feet above the anus to get sufficient pressure in the flow of water. The flow can be regulated by squeezing the tube with your fingers. Be sure that no air is left in the tube before inserting the nozzle into the anus. Use some vaseline on the nozzle to make insertion easier.

After emptying the bowel, a second enema, this time of one quart, may be taken. This larger enema will penetrate higher in the colon and accomplish a more thorough cleansing.

Warning: Enemas are intended only as a temporary measure during change-over period and are not intended to be a regular routine, or a habit. Although small one-pint enemas are perfectly harmless, larger enemas may slacken the bowel and damage the mucous membranes if used too frequently. When constipation is relieved and normal bowel movements achieved (as they will usually be on the Waerland-diet), then all enemas should be discontinued.

WAERLAND SYSTEM
IN PREVENTION AND CURE OF DISEASE

The Waerland system is basically a preventive health system. Waerland lectured and taught his health program to millions of healthy people with the purpose of improving their eating and living habits, preventing disease and achieving over-all better public health. But because of the fact that people generally are not interested in health until it starts to evade them, most people who listened to Waerland and adopted his ideas and his diet were sick people, in most cases incurably sick, given up by conventional medicine as hopeless cases. Thus the Waerland system became more a therapeutic than a prophylactic method, for which it was originally intended. Fortunately, a health system capable of protecting one's health and preventing disease is also generally capable of correcting disease and restoring health. Waerland's thereapeutic methods have now been applied in the treatment of many diseases in dozens of clinics and sanatoria in Europe and have proven to be very effective. Many remarkable cures are reported from time to time in various types of health literature from Europe.

ACTUAL REPORTED CASES OF CURES

This whole book could be filled with many remarkable cases of cures accomplished by the application of Waerland therapies. There is a book published by Ny Nord Förlag, in Sweden, called WAERLAND-DIET SAVED OUR LIVES, in which 50 ex-patients, who suffered with everything from cancer to psoriasis, tell about their cures with the help of Waerland therapies. The Swedish health magazine, Tidskrift för Hälsa, has reported hundreds of cases of cures accomplished by Waerland therapies in Swedish biological clinics. Here are a few cases to illustrate the point.

Mrs. Dorothy Olson, Höör, Sweden, suffered from severe hereditary asthma and was considered by doctors to be incurable. She also suffered from a bad case of migraine, which made her bedridden four to five days each month. She lived on frankfurters and coffee—up to 15 cups of coffee each day. After three months on a drastic Waerland program of fasting and strict diet, her asthma, as well as her migraine, were completely cured, never to come back.

Mrs. Irma Ericksson, Enshede, Sweden, suffered from chronic ulcerative colitis, a very serious bowel inflammation with bleeding ulcers. Her case was so bad that some days she had up to 40 stools. She suffered from this disease for 20 years, during which time she was treated by Sweden's best doctors. Once she stayed at Stockholm's St. Erik's Hospital for 12 months and was treated with many drugs, including cortisone. The cortisone treatment didn't help, but its side effect was a severe edema—she was swollen up with 20 pounds of extra water in her body, especially in her legs and face.

She started Waerland therapy with ten days of fasting, then had prescribed for her by a biologically-oriented doctor a special Dr. Ritters 10-day wheat diet. After this she started slowly with raw foods, with intermittent three-day fasts. After three months of treatments her ulcers were healed. After three more months all cramps and other symptoms were gone and her stomach and digestion were functioning quite normally. Examination and extensive tests at the hospital revealed that her ulcerative colitis was completely healed. Needless to say, her edema disappeared as well. Doctors considered her case so remarkable that they wanted her to come for periodic controls. Her case was studied and analyzed by the interns at the medical school. Now Mrs. Eriksson lives a normal life, works, exercises a lot, and skiis in the winter. Her diet consists mostly of yogurt, graham porridge (Molino*), raw vegetables, and especially lots of raw fruits of all kinds.

Mr. Knut Rosberg, Stockholm. The most remarkable case of cure by fasting is the case of Mr. Rosberg. He had suffered from gastric and duodenal ulcers for 22 years, off and on, and during the last two years was never without pain. Then, in 1954, he participated in the famous Swedish fast march, described in Chapter 2 of this book. It was a pure water fast for 10 days, during which the participants walked 300 miles from Gothenburg to Stockholm. The examination by X-rays one month after the fast march showed that he had no trace of an ulcer, not even a scar in his stomach and duodenum, where before the fast he had had as many as 15 ulcers.

Miss Monica Widlund, Eskilstuna, Sweden, was stricken by *arthritis* at a very early age. She was only two and a half years old. Doctors could not find the cause of the disease, nor were they able to help her during her many long stays at the hospitals. She was treated with cold injections and many drugs. In spite of the treatments she was becoming progressively worse. At the age of eight she was so bad that once she had to be carried home from school.

That year, 1954, she underwent biological therapy at the Brandal Clinic with two weeks of fasting followed by several weeks of raw food diet. She returned home completely restored to health. Nine years later, in 1963, she was interviewed and found to be in perfect health. She has never had a relapse and she now lives a perfectly normal life for a teenager—dances, plays and participates in sports. Biological therapies for arthritis which cured Monica Widlund are described in Chapter 9 of this book.

Mr. T. J. Andersson, Bandhagen, Sweden, had *high blood pressure,* a *ruptured disk* and was severely *overweight;* he was 5'7" and weighed 220 pounds.

He started with a one-month fast, then continued with a lacto-vegetarian diet. Later he adopted a strict raw vegetable diet, with no bread, cooked cereals or milk. After several months of alternating dieting and fasting he went down to his normal weight of 140 pounds, his blood pressure became normal, and he had only bad memories left of his ruptured disk. His favorite exercise is swimming. He swims every morning, even while fasting. Almost an invalid a few years ago, T. J. Andersson now swims 1,000 meters in 18–19 minutes!

Mrs. Greta Forsberg, Fors, Sweden, was born with *psoriasis*—a chronic skin disorder considered incurable by medical science. Her case was so bad that practically her entire body was affected, with the exception of her face and hands. She was treated at the Karolinska Hospital in Stockholm with vitamins A and B plus paraffin-baths.

The vitamin A treatment resulted in a temporary improvement, but didn't cure the problem.

On the advice of a Swedish chiropractor, she went to the clinic in Björkagården. There she received the usual biological treatments: one week's fasting, enemas, therapeutic baths, dry brushing, etc. The other important treatment was massage with almond oil each evening.

Improvement began immediately after the first two days of fasting. The typical white scaling diminished in quantity. After one week of fasting, about one-half of the affected area was improved. The improvement continued slowly during the special diet of vegetable foods, mostly raw fruits and vegetables.

"After two weeks I was so fantastically improved that I didn't believe my eyes. For the first time in my 46 years I could put on nylon stockings. Before I always had to use thick non-transparent stockings to hide my horrible looking legs," said Mrs. Forsberg.

Now Mrs. Forsberg is reported to be completely cured of her "incurable" psoriasis. On the advice of the Björkagården clinic, she fasts one week each month and continues with the vegetarian diet, although she admits that she is not always 100 percent consistent.

Her regular juice fasting is as follows:

- Breakfast: one glass of apricot juice and one glass of water.
- Lunch: one glass of natural grape juice and water.
- Dinner: a big bowl of vegetable broth.* The same before going to bed.
- Between "meals": pure, luke-warm water to make up a total liquid consumption during 24 hours of about three quarts.

Mrs. Elsa Eriksson, Lilla Essingen, Stockholm, was stricken with a *double breast cancer* 17 years ago, at the age of 40. The examination at the Karolinska Institute in Stockholm showed that there were distinct tumors in both breasts. Also the lymphatic glands were affected. Doctors insisted on an immediate operation the following week.

"I had no desire to be cut. I wanted to think it over. My brother informed me of the Waerland system and I went to visit a well-known naturopathic doctor in Stockholm," said Mrs. Eriksson. On his advice, she started her biological treatments which consisted of short fasts and a raw juice diet. After five weeks of fasting on water and juices she finally started with a raw food diet. About that time, she was called to Karolinska Institute for a final examination before the operation. After extensive examination, doctors, to their great surprise, could only declare that the tumors in both breasts had totally disappeared. There was no reason to operate!

Mrs. Eriksson's case is well-documented with extensive examinations by renowned doctors. She visited the same hospital three to five times each year for the next five years for examination. Each time the examination revealed that the tumors had disappeared and that her health condition was good. Sixteen years after the cancer was diagnosed, she was still, at the age of 56, in perfect health and free from cancer. Naturally she faithfully continues with the diet which saved her from the cancer operation.

6

How a Low-Animal-Protein Diet
Can Improve Your Health and
Help Prevent Premature Aging

When I recently met Dr. Karl-Otto Aly, a prominent Swedish doctor, upon his return from a lecture tour in the United States and asked, "What was the one most memorable impression of this trip," he said:

"The American high-protein craze! Not only the general public, but even the so-called health enthusiasts are so thoroughly brainwashed on the question of protein in their diet that, to my mind, this factor alone may be held to a great degree responsible for the deplorable state of health of the American people—in addition, of course, to the American over-processed, chemicalized and devitalized foods."

Dr. Aly told me that after his lectures people would come to the stage and look closely at his face to see if he didn't have rouge on it. They just couldn't believe that a man could look so healthy and robust without eating meat. They kept asking him, "But where do you get your proteins?"

The absolute maxim of any respectable American health system is its *high-protein* requirement. Yet, practically all the top men in the European health field are unanimous in their endorsement of a low-protein diet, particularly a low-animal-protein diet, as the diet most conducive to good health and long life! Empirical evidence in support of low-protein as against high-protein intake is equally impressive.

HOW THE HIGH-PROTEIN MYTH ORIGINATED

The scientific fact that our bodies are made up mostly of proteins may be largely responsible for the high-protein myth. But powerful American advertising must have played the decisive role in building up the high-protein cult. There is no money in advertising health. But there seem to be huge economic interests involved in promoting the high-protein diet.

You are subjected to continuous, never-ending high-protein propaganda every day of your life. Periodical reports of "scientific research," naturally sponsored by the livestock, dairy or meat packing industry, see to it that you'll never forget your need for "lots of proteins." You read this in the medical syndicated columns of your daily newspaper; you read it in popular health magazines and health books on nutrition by "experts" and "authorities." You have been taught this in your grade school, your Home-Ec course in high school, and your nutrition classes in college. You have been fed this propaganda and geared for the high-protein cult for decades, from all possible directions, even roadside billboards and "beef for health" stickers on automobile bumpers! You are advised to eat lots of meat, fish, eggs, and milk to get as much protein as possible. In fact, you are basically told that you can never get too much protein in your diet.

HOW MUCH PROTEIN DO YOU NEED?

It is true, of course, that your body is built mostly of proteins. It is also true that proteins are vital nutritive elements and are absolutely necessary in your nutrition. Twenty percent, or more in some vital organs, of a cell's composition is made up of protein. Since your body is constantly renewing and repairing its cells, you need lots of protein in your diet to supply all the needed amino acids, or "building blocks" for these repairs and the rebuilding of cells.

But how much is "lots"? 70, 100, 150, 200, or more grams a day, as advocated by many "experts"?

The growing number of responsible nutritionists in various

parts of the world are coming to the realization that our present beliefs on the protein question are outdated and that the actual need for protein in human nutrition is far below that which has long been considered necessary. Furthermore, recent research has demonstrated that vegetable proteins, formerly believed to be incomplete and inferior to animal proteins, *are actually biologically as good or better than animal proteins;* and that good health can be sustained *on a lesser amount of raw vegetable protein than animal protein.*

First, a Finnish scientist, Dr. V. O. Siven, showed that our daily need of protein was only approximately 30 grams. Then the famous American scientist, Dr. R. Chittenden, arrived at similar results after long and extensive experiments with sportsmen and soldiers. He found that 35–50 grams of protein a day are sufficient to keep the nitrogen balance in the body. (This is the usual criterion for determining the protein requirement.) Dr. Chittenden has also shown that physical performance in sports and heavy strenuous work is *better on a low protein diet.* In 1946, Dr. D. M. Hegsted of Harvard University proved that the average person's need for protein is 32.4 grams a day, if he uses mixed proteins from vegetable origin. If one-third of the protein intake is from milk, then the minimum protein requirement will be as low as 27.1 grams a day. The world-famous Swedish nutritionist, Dr. Ragnar Berg, whose works on nutrition are used as textbooks in many medical schools, did extensive research on protein needs and came to the conclusion that 30 grams of protein in the daily diet is a generous allowance. Finally, Dr. William C. Rose has shown that only 20 grams a day of mixed proteins (of which only about ⅔ are so-called "complete") are sufficient for our needs.

Studies made in Germany by Professor K. Eimer showed that the performance of athletes improved after they switched from a daily 100-gram animal protein diet to a 50-gram vegetable protein diet. Japanese research showed that 25–30 grams of protein a day are sufficient to sustain good health.

Taking into consideration the great variation in protein need of each individual and the extra demands under conditions of stress or disease, a generous conclusion would be that 50–60 grams of protein daily, derived 75–80 percent from vegetable sources, are sufficient for optimum health. Proteins in excess of this amount are *not needed by the body and are only burned as fuel for energy, and as an energy food proteins are inferior to carbohydrates and fats.* The digestion of proteins in excess of this actual need leaves toxic metabolic waste products which contribute to self-intoxication and disease.

PROTEIN FADS AND FALLACIES

In addition to the high-protein diet fallacy there are many other protein fads and fallacies, such as:

1. *"You should eat lots of proteins every day!"* The fact is that your body can exist without *any* food, and, consequently, *without any protein*, for weeks and months, as, for example, in the case of complete therapeutic fasting. (See Chapter 2.) And this not only is not harmful but has evident health benefits. It is a general observation that the protein level of the blood (serum albumin reading) of fasting patients remains constant and normal during the whole fasting period, in spite of the fact that no protein is consumed. The reason for this is that proteins in your body are in the so-called *dynamic state:* that means that they are constantly changed from one stage to another, being decomposed and resynthesized from blood plasma amino acids. (This phenomenon, which is so little understood as yet, may help solve some of the protein cult mystery.) Thus, the body is using and re-using the same proteins again and again where they are needed.

This proves that you do not need to eat high-protein meals *every day,* although your body does need protein each day. You will improve your health by eating a low-protein vegetable and fruit diet several days a week. And you can do it safely and without worrying about "where do I get my proteins?"

2. *"You need meat for proteins!"* The most commonly asked question when meat-eaters talk with vegetarians or lacto-vegetarians is a "but where do you get your proteins?"

The answer is that since proteins are such vital and important nutritive substances, our Creator in his infinite wisdom has made them a part of virtually every natural food available to man. Every plant, every vegetable, every fruit, every seed or nut contains some protein. It is practically impossible to eat a natural food without eating *some* protein. The fact is that it is virtually impossible to get too few proteins on any diet, unless you are on a starvation diet. But it is not only possible, but very likely that you will develop a serious deficiency of vitamins and vital substances on the one-sided diet of meat, potatoes and bread so common in the United States. A meatless diet of raw fruits and vegetables, potatoes, whole bread, milk and cheese, nuts and beans will not only supply all the proteins you need, but is also rich in all the vitamins, minerals, and enzymes essential for optimum health.

The protein quality in some of the vegetables sources is even superior to the meat protein, as in the case of protein from soybeans, some nuts (cashews, almonds), potatoes and green vegetables. You may not know it, but plain old potatoes are a good source of complete proteins. You have been made to believe that potatoes are a pure starch food, but they contain large amounts of complete proteins, biologically comparable to the protein in eggs.[1] In some experiments, men lived three to six years with potatoes as the only protein source and maintained excellent health and performed hard work. In the average German diet, ten percent of the daily protein requirement is derived from potatoes.

Much recent research shows that your body's protein requirement is lowered *if the protein is obtained from raw vegetable sources.* Professor Eimer in Germany showed that athletes, switched from 100 grams of animal proteins a day to 50 grams of raw vegetable proteins, grew stronger and improved their records.[2] Also a Japanese researcher, Dr. M. Kuratsune, has demonstrated that 22–30 grams of raw vegetable protein a day were sufficient to keep him and his wife in good health.[3]

The foremost scientific authority on nutrition today is the International Society for Research on Nutrition and Vital Substances. Their recommendation in regard to protein reads: "The conception of the classical and late-classical nutrition theory that animal proteins are more valuable than plant proteins, *can no longer be accepted.* Today we know that the order of rank of proteins is generally dependent on their amino-gram and not on their origin." They also state: "Each plant protein contains *all the exogenous-essential amino acids.*"[4]

3. *"Only complete proteins can satisfy your protein needs."* This is another common but fallacious statement made in support of "complete" meat proteins. Such foods as soybeans, sesame seeds, many nuts, millet, potatoes, and green vegetables all contain complete proteins, as good or better than meat proteins, without meat's undesirable side effects.

Furthermore, it is a proven physiological fact that several foods with incomplete proteins will complement one another if eaten at the same time, and thus render their *total protein* biologically complete. For example: although wheat protein is lacking in some of the essential amino acids, a cheese sandwich on whole wheat bread will be a complete protein meal, with the cheese complementing the wheat and supplying the missing amino acids. Beans and tortillas, eaten with some vegetables, also make a complete protein meal, although beans and corn are not complete separately. The Journal of the American Medical Association reported that protein, which is derived in proportion up to two-thirds from plant origin, adequately supplies all the protein needed for normal growth and sustenance of health.[5]

Thus the notion that only foods with all the essential amino acids can satisfy your protein need is fallacious.

4. *"You need animal proteins for strength!"* This fallacy will be difficult to disprove, because steak lovers just love to think that meat gives them strength. The truth is, however, exactly the opposite. And this is proven in scientific experiments over and over again.

Professor Irving Fisher made comparative studies of meat-eating Yale athletes with non-meat-eating vegetarians, doctors and assistants from the Battle Creek Sanatorium. The following tests were given to two groups. First, the men were to hold their arms outstretched as long as possible. Only two of the meat-eaters reached 15 minutes, while 22 of the 32 vegetarians were able to achieve this. None of the meat-eaters, but 15 vegetarians, reached a half-hour. Nine of these reached one hour, four two hours, and one three hours and 20 minutes. The second test was deep knee bends. Only a few of the meat-eaters were able to make more than 300–400 knee bends. One vegetarian made 1,800, one 2,400, and one 5,000. Dr. Fisher concluded that the protein content in the diet was responsible for the difference in endurance and stamina. In his continuous experiments, he further lowered the protein intake of the persons under study and noticed that a 20 percent reduction in protein increased their endurance 33 percent.[6]

Even studies made by Dr. R. Chittenden of Yale University have shown that endurance increases with a lower protein intake. His experiments with professors, students, soldiers and athletes proved that muscle strength and endurance reaches its peak on about one-third of the usual protein intake. His explanation of this phenomenon was that the protein metabolism results in the higher blood content of uric acid, urea, and purines, and that these have a toxic, paralyzing effect on muscles and nerves. This may explain the observation made by westerners in Hong Kong harbour, where the little Chinese coolies carry 200-pound rice bags all day long, eating nothing but rice and vegetables. Asked why don't they eat meat, one of them said, "If I ate meat I would not be able to carry these bags all day long." The great Australian swimming champion, Murray Rose, Olympic Gold Medal winner for several years, has never tasted meat in his life—he has been a 100 percent vegetarian since birth. Most of the Japanese endurance swimmers eat little or no meat. You may also remember Horace Braby, a young South African athlete who won over all his meat-eating competitors on a meatless diet; or the remarkable victories of New Zealander John Marshall in 1956 in the long-distance swimming contest; or Bill Pickering "who crossed the English Channel and on his arrival was able to run up the beach"—all on diets without meat but rich in raw vegetable foods.[7]

WHAT'S WRONG WITH THE HIGH PROTEIN DIET?

The greatest fault with high-protein diet is that your body cannot store any appreciable amount of protein. It uses only what is needed and the rest is burned up as energy or deposited in the body in the form of fat. As energy food, however, protein is inferior to carbohydrates or fats. The digestion of animal protein causes building of certain toxins. The nitrogen is transformed to urea or uric acid and, as in the case of sluggish metabolism and inefficient elimination, it is deposited in body tissues. This causes self-poisoning, or autointoxication.

A high animal protein diet also causes intestinal putrefaction and constipation. In addition, meat contains many toxins of metabolic origin, which remain in the tissues when the animal is killed. These toxins lay a further strain on the eliminative organs, particularly on the kidneys. Furthermore, most meats these days are loaded with antibiotics and other drugs used in animal feeding to speed the fattening process. The following drugs are used for this purpose: penicillin, streptomycin, tetracycline, aureomycin, terramycin, bacitracin, chlortetra cycline, oxytetracycline tylosin, and arsenic. It is estimated that 75 percent of all the beef sold in America today has been fed rations containing dietylstilbestrol, a synthetic hormone used to fatten livestock. It is known to be possibly carcinogenic. So if you eat lots of meat, you can be reasonably sure that you are receiving a heavy dose of this hormone each day, since much of it remains in the carcass after the animal is killed. According to drug manuals, stilbestrol can also cause edema, skin eruption, uterine bleeding, congestive heart failure, loss of libido in males, and many other disorders.

Most of the natural foods, such as grains, seeds, vegetables, and legumes are all-round foods, composed of well-balanced amounts of carbohydrates, proteins, fats, vitamins, minerals, enzymes and other vital substances. Meat, with the exception of some organ meats, is a one-sided protein food, practically void of most vitamins and low in mineral content.

A diet high in protein causes biochemical imbalance in the system, especially in respect to vitamins. It has been experimentally proven that vitamin B deficiency, especially deficiency in vitamin B_6, can be caused by prolonged high animal protein diet.[8] Recent research by the doctors at the Vascular Research Laboratory in Brooklyn indicates that the meat-eating habit could be a cause of widespread arteriosclerosis and heart disease.[9] And, of course, it is common knowledge these days that meat, no matter how lean it is, contains a large percentage of saturated fats loaded with cholesterol, which raise the cholesterol content of the blood and may lead to heart disease. Currently, a high protein diet is under suspicion as a possible culprit in many degenerative diseases, including arthritis. At the recent annual Rheumatism Foundation meeting, Dr. Donald A. Gerber, professor of medicine at New York State University, stated that the development of rheumatoid arthritis could be caused by a defect in body chemistry which interferes with the metabolism of protein. He then suggested that a low protein diet may provide the answer to sufferers from arthritis.[10]

EMPIRICAL EVIDENCE

There is no better way than the empirical way to prove any given nutritional theory. Our knowledge of intricate body chemistry and metabolism is rudimental and new facts are discovered daily. But if we can put the theory into practice and see what results it has produced through centuries or even millenniums of use, then it is worth more than bookshelves full of scientific reasoning.

The secret of the Hunzakuts

There is one particular nation which is generally considered "the healthiest people on earth"—the Hunza people. First "discovered" by Sir Robert McCarrison, famous British physician, in the beginning of this century, Hunza has been visited since that time by many researchers, attracted there by the Hunza people's remarkably good health and freedom from all diseases common to the "civilized world." Hunza is located in the Himalayas and is a quiet, isolated kingdom of about 25,000 inhabitants.

Cancer, heart diseases, diabetes, rheumatic diseases and many other diseases common in western countries are unknown in Hunza. Do not try to discount this by the usual "they-don't-have-proper-diagnosis" argument. A very competent physician, Dr. McCarrison, lived among them for 11 years and tried hard to find traces of these diseases. "They know no sickness," he said. They live up to 90, 100 and over 100 years of age; are virile, strong and active long after they reach the usual three score and ten.

The researchers who studied Hunza agree that *their diet is the major factor in their unusual health and longevity.* Primitive life and healthful mountainous climate are, of course, contributing factors; but some other tribes in the same area, but with different eating habits, do not demonstrate nearly as good health as the Hunzakuts do. The Hunza diet is a *high natural carbohydrate—low animal protein diet!* Their staple foods are grains, such as wheat, barley, millet, and buckwheat; fruits, mostly apricots, apples, and grapes; assorted vegetables, generally eaten raw; and very little milk, largely goat milk. They eat few eggs and very little meat, only on festive occasions and not more than once a month. Needless to say, because of their isolated and inaccessible position in the Himalaya mountains, they have no access to refined, civilized foods made from white flour, white sugar, canned foods, etc. The Hunzas are a living proof that an unrefined, simple diet, rich in natural carbohydrates and low in animal proteins is superior to our over-refined, devitalized protein-rich diet.

Yemenites

A few years ago, a tribe of Semitic origin was discovered in the mountains of Yemen. Several thousand people were living high in the mountains in an area isolated from the rest of the world for over

2,000 years, with customs and living and eating habits of the pre-Christian era. Of course, the sensational news was publicized in the world press. Many scientists from all over the world immediately rushed to Yemen to study these people, their way of life, their health conditions, eating habits, etc. They discovered that these Yemenites were specimens of perfect health who lived to a very old age and knew practically no diseases. And what did they eat? You've guessed it! Yes, theirs was a *low animal protein—high natural carbohydrate diet!*

Russians

Russians are known for their endurance and good health. They have seven times more centenarians per million than the United States. Russians are a low-protein people. Their staples are black whole-grain bread with lots of vegetables (mostly cabbage, onions and potatoes) and grains like millet and buckwheat. Russian sour black rye bread,* borsch (vegetable soup) and kasha* (millet or buckwheat porridge) are world-famous. They seldom eat meat more than once a week. 74.5 percent of their protein need is derived from vegetable sources and only 25.5 percent from animal sources (as compared with the United States figures of 29 percent vegetable and 71 percent animal!). Of course, the greatest number of Russia's 21,000 centenarians are vegetarians, or nearly vegetarians. During the war many of their armed units lived on meatless diets for months and demonstrated remarkable stamina and endurance.

Bulgarians

Bulgarians are among the healthiest races in Europe. They are, along with the Scandinavians, the tallest people in Europe and they possess great vitality and longevity. There are more centenarians in Bulgaria than in any other civilized country. They are known to retain the characteristics of youth to an advanced age. The virility of their "old" men is legendary. According to the 1930 census, Bulgarians had 1,600 centenarians to every million of population as

---

* Wherever they appear, asterisks (*) indicate that the recipe or direction cited may be found in Chapter 16.

compared to nine persons of 100 years old or older per million in the
United States.

The diet of the Bulgarians consists largely of black bread
(mostly whole rye and barley), vegetables and soured milk in the
form of yogurt* or kefir.* They eat relatively little meat.

Seventh-Day Adventists

A grand-scale scientific evidence supporting the low animal
protein diet is presented in the health statistics from a religious
group, the Seventh-Day Adventists.

A study conducted by Dr. Frank R. Lemon and Dr. Richard T.
Walden, of the Loma Linda School of Medicine, reveals that the
Seventh-Day Adventists, as a group, have better health and live
longer than the general population. Their rate of lung cancer is
practically zero, 1000 percent or ten times less than among the
general population. This is true even among those Adventists who
live in the heavy-smogged Los Angeles area! The rate of coronary
disease among them is 40 percent less than in the general population.
Studies reveal low mortality and low morbidity among Seventh-Day
Adventists from all cancers of the respiratory tract and esophagus,
emphysema and bronchitis, and from coronary artery disease.

The Seventh-Day Adventist mortality rate from all causes is two
times lower, and from respiratory diseases four times lower, than
among the general population.

Now, here we have an extraordinarily remarkable scientific
study made by reputable medical men and reported in the Journal of
the American Medical Association, which shows that a certain group
of people, living in the United States seemingly under the same
conditions as the rest of us, possesses vastly superior health. Wouldn't
this study be worth looking into in our multibillion-dollar quest for
ways of improving the catastrophic state of our health?

The answer to the superior health of the Seventh-Day Adventists lies in the health program advocated by their Church. They look
upon their bodies as the Temples of the Spirit and, as such, keep it
clean and in good repair. They are lacto-vegetarians; they eat no
meat. They do not smoke, drink no alcohol, nor do they use coffee,
tea or other caffein-containing beverages such as cola drinks. They
are also advised to abstain from the consumption of sugar and refined
starches. A recent study made by the Colorado State Health Depart-

ment reveals that Seventh-Day Adventist children have about 50 percent fewer cavities than the other children in the area.

SUMMARY

I hope that the evidence presented in this chapter, both scientific and empirical, is sufficient to show that it is not the high protein diet, but the *high natural carbohydrate—low animal protein diet* that is the diet most conducive to optimum health, maximum vitality, and long life.

To be sure, you need good proteins in your diet. Proteins are essential for the proper functioning of all your vital organs and for the rebuilding and repair of your cells. But you must see that your diet does not contain too much animal protein. A high animal protein diet may cause such disturbances as overacidity, intestinal putrefaction, constipation, uric acid accumulation in the blood and tissues, high blood pressure, high blood cholesterol level, obesity, etc.; and it may be a major predisposing factor in the development of such diseases as arthritis and heart disease. Studies have shown that a low protein vegetarian diet can prevent 97 percent of coronary occlusions.[11] Other tests have shown that the amount of the essential amino acids cystine and tyrosine in the diets of vegetarians exceeded twice their minimum requirement and compared favorably to nonvegetarians.[12]

A diet rich in raw fruits and vegetables, whole grains, seeds, nuts, beans, raw unpasteurized milk and milk products such as cheese, yogurt and dry milk powder, and fortified with wheat germ, brewer's yeast and cold-pressed vegetable oils, will supply you not only with all the essential vitamins, minerals, enzymes, trace elements, and other vital substances, but with all the necessary proteins as well.

High natural carbohydrate—low animal protein diet holds the greatest potential for optimum health, vitality and extended longevity.

This is not a theory, hypothesis or wishful thinking. This is an established scientific fact. The Scientific Council of the International Society for Research on Nutrition and Vital Substances—the most objective, independent and qualified scientific authority on nutrition today—made the following recommendation for a completely balanced diet of optimum nutrition for optimum health:

"A human being needs:
- for the undisturbed physiological functioning of his organism,
- for sufficient vitality and energy to carry out his daily responsibilities,
- and for building up of optimum health and prevention of diseases of old age,

a complete diet of whole foods with the following characteristics:
- natural foods, free from harmful additives,
- an adequate supply of vital substances (vitamins, minerals, enzymes, proteins, fatty acids, trace elements, etc.),
- a moderate supply of calories and energy-producing foods such as refined carbohydrates,
- a lacto-vegetarian diet of fresh foods (diet of whole grains, vegetables, fruits, seeds, nuts, and milk and milk products)."

HOW TO PLAN YOUR LOW-ANIMAL-PROTEIN DIET FOR BETTER HEALTH AND PREVENTION OF DISEASE

In practical terms, for the profitable application of the information in this chapter and the assurance of optimal health and the prevention of disease and premature aging, abide by the following rules with regard to protein in your diet:

1. Eliminate, or cut drastically, all meat from your diet. If you insist on animal protein, ocean fish and eggs are preferable to meat.

2. Raw, unpasteurized milk and milk products such as soured milk,* yogurt,* kefir,* and homemade cottage cheese* are good, wholesome sources of complete proteins. Use them to complement the protein sources of vegetable origin, such as:

3. Whole grains, seeds, lentils and nuts. Soybeans are particularly rich in complete proteins, which are superior to meat protein. Sesame seeds, millet and sunflower seeds are also great protein sources. Millet and buckwheat can be used to make delicious cereals.* Sesame seeds are nutritious and delicious in the form of homemade Halvah.* Sunflower seeds should be eaten raw, as they are, or ground and sprinkled on fruit salads or other dishes. Whole wheat and rye breads* from freshly-ground flour are rich in good proteins; so are Kruska,* Molino* and other whole grain cereals, particularly in combination with milk. All kinds of beans and peas should be used liberally in your diet; their proteins are not complete, but nevertheless they are high-grade proteins which are rendered

complete in combination with other foods. Nuts are excellent sources of protein, especially almonds, cashews and peanuts. Nuts should always be eaten raw, not roasted.

4. Many readers do not know how to use all these seeds and nuts, especially older people who do not have good teeth to chew them raw. Here's good advise: buy a tiny seed grinder! Health food stores or drug stores usually have several varieties to offer at prices from $9.00 to $12.00. In a few seconds you can grind to a fine powder any of the grains, seeds, or nuts and use them conveniently mixed with other foods or blended with milk or juices. Of course, they also could be liquefied in an ordinary blender, or osterizer, mixed with water, milk or juice.

5. Do not ignore vegetables as a protein source. Green leafy vegetables contain complete proteins of the highest biological value. Potatoes are a very good source of complete proteins. Potatoes should be boiled or baked whole with their jackets on.

6. Fortify your diet with such high-protein sources as wheat germ and brewer's yeast. Two or three tablespoons of wheat germ a day will give you a large amount of good protein in addition to a virtual gold mine of vitamins and minerals. A half cup of raw wheat germ contains 24 grams of protein, more than in a quarter-pound of beef! A pound of raw wheat germ, which costs about 30 cents, gives you over 100 grams of protein. Brewer's yeast, or food yeast, is an even better source of protein than wheat germ. Two tablespoons of yeast contain as much protein as half a cup of wheat germ, or more than a quarter-pound hamburger.

7

The Healing Power of Raw Fruit and Vegetable Juices

American readers need no introduction to juices. The United States can take credit for the popularization of juice both as a food and as a drink. Juices of countless kinds and descriptions form a major part of the food processing industry. Just walk to any supermarket and you will see whole departments of long shelves full of various brands of juices and drinks. You'll find juices in gallon jars, in tin cans, in glass bottles, and in waxed cartons. You may have your juice fresh, frozen, canned, concentrated, mixed, reconstituted, synthetic, sugar-added, natural, colored—have your pick! You can buy it at your favorite food store, get it from the automatic dispenser, buy it at the corner drug store or garage, or have it delivered to your doorstep each morning by your milkman. Almost all Americans drink juice for breakfast, lunch, and dinner. We are, without question, the biggest juice drinkers in the world!

Although the popularity of juice is based on the premise that it is good for your health—and for this reason many a mother forces orange juice down the throats of her kids each morning—it does not seem to have been doing any good for the health of the American people. It seems that we are much sicker now than a generation or two back, prior to the juice drinking fad.

The explanation of this paradox is simple. The kind of juices most Americans drink not only lack health-giving properties, but may, in addition, be hazardous to health. Because of extensive processing, heating, chemical treatments, synthetic artificial colorings and flavorings, sugar or artificial sweeteners, and additions of many toxic preservatives, the juices or the so-called juice drinks you buy at your supermarket today bear no resemblance to the juices which were originally meant to be health-giving beverages—fresh, raw, natural juices. Just read the labels on the cans and you'll see what I mean!

So let's make this thing clear once and for all: the only juices which can be considered as health-giving, or conducive to good health and well-being, and can be recommended for the therapeutic use in the healing of disease or as a preventive measure in maintaining good health, are *fresh, raw, natural juices, prepared immediately before drinking from fresh fruits, berries, vegetables, and green plants*. Such juices you won't find at the usual kind of supermarket.

JUICE—FOOD OR MEDICINE?

The best way to consume fresh fruits and vegetables is to eat them, not to drink them. By eating raw fruits and vegetables you not only supply your body with all the health-giving vital nutritive elements they contain, but also provide your digestive organs with sufficient amounts of bulk or roughage (the cellulose), which is imperative for the effective digestion and assimilation of food and the elimination of wastes.

When you try to determine the healthfulness of a certain food or substance, your first question should be *"is it natural?"* Nature has provided ample amounts and great varieties of natural foods for man; foods which need no preparation, refinement, processing or concentration. According to this criterion, juice is not natural food in the full sense of the word. It is a highly concentrated and fragmentary food, which can be used very effectively as a medicine in treatment of certain diseases, but is largely unnecessary as a regular part of the daily diet of healthy individuals. Yes, certain juices may even be harmful if consumed in large amounts and over long periods of time.

There is much evidence against, for example, the indiscriminate use of citrus juices. Eating citrus fruits moderately is a healthy habit, but drinking citrus juices regularly may be the cause of many disorders. British researchers have shown that drinking fruit juices will cause loss of calcium from the teeth, with consequent erosion of the teeth.[1] From the biological point of view, the unbalanced concentration of nutrients in juices can be detrimental to the biochemistry of the body. If some of the foods are juiced and the others are consumed whole, certain nutrients could be over-supplied, while the others are under-supplied. Also, it should be kept in mind that all the nutrients present in whole foods cannot be juiced out; some of them will still remain in the pulp. This is bound to cause a chemical imbalance and metabolic disorder in the system.

Therefore, the general principle is that you should eat your food, not drink it. Small occasional additions of freshly-made juices would naturally do no harm, and perhaps would even do some good. My objections are against using large amounts of fruit juices every day for long periods of time.

The above objections are directed to people in good health. As I stated before, the rightful place for raw juices is in the treatment of disease. Juice as a medicine is one of the major biological agents in the treatment of almost every disease. Many outstanding medical and naturopathic practitioners have used juices in their therapeutic programs with remarkable success. In the famous Dr. Max Gerson's cancer clinic fresh juices were a main therapeutic measure. All European biological clinics use raw juices in their programs of treatment. As I have mentioned in Chapter 2, practically all fasts in European clinics are now done with juices.

RAW JUICE THERAPY

One of the greatest authorities on using raw juices for therapeutic purposes is Georg Lányi, M.D., from Gothenburg, Sweden. Dr. Lányi served for many years on the staff of the famous Buchinger clinic in Germany, where juice fasting is done by thousands of patients each year. He has had extensive experience with using different juices and their combinations for specific ailments. Much of the following information is taken from his illuminative article *Raw Juices Instead of Drugs*.[2]

The favorable effect of raw juices in treatment of diseases, particularly in combination with fasting, is attributed to the following physiological facts:

• Vital minerals, vitamins and trace elements present in juices are assimilated almost 100 percent from the digestive tract.

• They provide an alkaline surplus to balance the acids which are in large quantity in the blood and tissues during fasting.

These factors have a stimulating and exhilarating effect on the detoxicating, cleansing and healing processes. The amount of juices, therefore, should be carefully controlled in accordance with specific needs, just as it is with any other kind of medication. The total juice intake in 24 hours should be between a pint and a quart and a half, never more. It is advisable in most cases that one half of the daily intake is fruit juice, the other half vegetable juice.

The most effective way to use juices for therapeutic purpose is in the form of a juice fast, as described in Chapter 2 of this book.

The shortest juice fast is seven to eight days, the longest three to four weeks, and sometimes even longer. Fasting for one week is usually sufficient for prophylactic purposes; that is, when people in relatively good health fast regularly to cleanse the system of accumulated impurities and to give the digestive and other organs time to rest and thus restore their functions to peak performance—rather like the servicing and tune-up that we have on our automobiles. The length of the therapeutic juice fast should be determined by the experienced practitioner.

Here is a list of minerals, trace elements, vitamins, enzymes, coloring substances and other elements present in specific juices, with their prophylactic and therapeutic importance.

Minerals in raw juices

CALCIUM: MDR† 0.8 gram. Present mostly in lemons, tangerines, elderberries, nettles, kohlrabi, watercress and turnip tops. Needed for bone formation, prevents inflammations and has a favorable preventive influence on tendency for hemorrhage.

POTASSIUM: MDR 0.5–1.0 g. Present in grapes, tangerines, lemons, spinach, potatoes, kale and most green leafy vegetables. Important for nerve and muscle function.

SODIUM: MDR 0.2–0.4 g. Present mostly in cherries, peaches, beets, dandelions, carrots, celery, and tomatoes.

MAGNESIUM: MDR 0.3 g. Present mostly in elderberries, raspberries, lemons, endive and nettles. Soothes nervous irritability, is important for muscle action

---

† Minimum Daily Requirement

and is indispensable in mineral and general metabolism.

PHOSPHORUS: MDR 0.9 g. Present in grapes, raspberries, tangerines, spinach, watercress and kale. Plays vital part in bone formation.

SULPHUR: MDR 0.3 g. Present mostly in black and red currants, spinach, watercress and kale. Important in liver and skin-cell metabolism.

IRON: MDR 12 mg. Present in red and black currants, raspberries, spinach, apricots, parsley and nettles. Vital for cell oxygenation as a constituent of hemoglobin.

Trace elements in raw juices

There is no exact information available in regard to the precise needs of these elements in human nutrition, but it has been established that deficiency in these substances can result in diseases in humans, animals and plants.

COPPER: Present in black and red currants, kale, potatoes and asparagus. Helps in iron absorption.

MANGANESE: Present in strawberries, apricots, oranges, green lettuce, spinach and kale. Involved, among other things, in reproductive processes.

ZINC: Present in apples, pears, kale, lettuce and asparagus. Needed for nerves. The healthy function of the prostate gland is dependent upon a sufficient amount of zinc in the diet.

COBALT: Present in apples and yellow onions. Assists in hemoglobin production.

FLUORINE: Present in black currants, cherries, spinach and carrots. There is a great controversy as to its need in nutrition.

IODINE: Present in oranges and spinach. Participates in metabolism through the thyroid gland.

SILICIC ACID: Present in strawberries, grapes, lettuce and carrots. Constitutes an important part of bone composition and is especially beneficial during healing processes.

Vitamins, enzymes, coloring substances, etc. in raw juices

Vitamin A: Does not occur in vitamin form in vegetables or fruits, but as a provitamin, *carotene,* which is transformed by the body into vitamin A. It is present mostly in carrots, green and red peppers, rose hips and oranges. Absorption of vitamin A into the digestive tract can be aided by the addition of linseed oil (flaxseed oil) or sesame seed oil to the juices.

Vitamin B$_1$: Present mostly in grapefruit, spinach, dandelion.

Vitamin B$_2$: Present mostly in parsley, spinach and kale.

Vitamin B$_3$: Present mostly in parsley, potatoes and asparagus.

Vitamin B$_5$: Present mostly in cabbage, cauliflower, strawberries, grapefruit and oranges.

Vitamin B$_6$: Present mostly in pears, spinach, potatoes, lemons and carrots.

Folic acid: Present mostly in spinach, parsley, potatoes and oranges.

Biotin: Present mostly in cauliflower, spinach, lettuce and grapefruit.

Inositol: Present mostly in oranges, grapefruit, cauliflower, kale and onions.

Vitamin C: The most known and universally used vitamin. The need is much greater than the tables usually recommend, especially during all kinds of infection, even chronic infections. Present in black currants, citrus fruits, green peppers, nettles, parsley and, most of all, in rose hips.

Vitamin K: Present in nettles, spinach and cabbage.

Vitamin P: Present mostly in grapes, oranges, black currants, rose hips, plums and green peppers.

Vitamin E: Present in cold-pressed vegetable oils, especially in wheat germ oil.

Enzymes: Many important enzymes are present in raw juices. Enzymes are made inactive by heating over 60° C.

Coloring substances: Yellow, red, green and blue coloring substances in all shades and intensities are present in large quantities in raw juices. They are vitally important from a therapeutic point of view. According to Dr. Georg Lányi, they increase production of red blood corpuscles, influence digestive and assimilative processes, and take part in the metabolism of proteins and cholesterol, etc.[8]

In addition, raw juices contain the hormone-like substances, the "vegetable hormones," and antibiotic substances, which are, for example, present in garlic, onions, radishes, tomatoes, etc.

WHAT DISEASES CAN BE TREATED
WITH RAW JUICE THERAPY?

First, it must be emphasized that every case is different and therefore all treatments must be adapted for every individual case. Especially with regard to fasting, the patient's physical and mental condition should be taken into consideration. It can vary from year to year in the same person! The suggestions given below are, therefore, to be considered only in a very general sense. If you suffer from a serious ailment it is best to consult a biologically-oriented doctor on the advisability of undertaking raw juice therapy.

Infectious diseases

The response to raw juice therapy in all forms of infectious disease is excellent. Tonsillitis also responds well.

The juices of black currants, lemons, oranges, elderberries, beets, carrots, tomatoes, watercress, onion, garlic (in very small doses), and rose hips are useful in the treatment of infectious diseases.

Stomach disorders

Gastric catarrh, or *gastritis,* responds well to the therapy of raw juices of carrots, tomatoes, celery and potatoes. Cabbage juice (vitamin U) is considered specifically curative for gastric catarrh and stomach ulcers. *Liver and gall bladder* diseases (gall bladder inflammation) are best treated with the juice of grapes, carrots, and beets with small additions of juice from dandelions and radishes. Pear juice has been found very effective in the treatment of gall bladder diseases and gall stones. Diseases of the *small intestine* and all forms of constipation can be improved by raw juice therapy. Garlic exerts a cleansing effect on the bowels and is beneficial in cases of excessive gas. The juice of yellow onions has a similar, but milder, effect. These juices can be used in small amounts, one teaspoon or one tablespoon at a time.

For *chronic constipation* the following juices are recommended: nettles, spinach, watercress, garlic, yellow onions, black radish, and dandelion in addition to the milder juices of carrots, cucumber, tomatoes, red beets, and celery. Sauerkraut juice cleans bowels well, but some patients are troubled with gas when they use sauerkraut.

Of the fruit juices, apple and lemon are recommended in stomach disorders. Blueberries are excellent in cases of catarrhs; they are also the best medicine for diarrhea.

Blood and heart diseases

Variations in the amounts of red blood cells can be treated with juices. "Thick" blood, *polycythemia,* will be thinner after two or three weeks of juice therapy. The treatment can be repeated several times. For "thin" blood, *anemia,* spinach and nettle juices are effective. They are rich in iron and chlorophyll, the green coloring matter of the leaves. These juices can be added to carrot juice in amounts of approximately three to four ounces a day.

The dark colored juices of grapes, beets and blueberries help increase the production of red blood cells.[4] Blood circulation is also improved by the juices, mainly because of the favorable strengthening effect they have on the tiny blood capillaries.

For disorders in the normal *heart function,* juices of hawthorn berries and garlic can be added to the other milder juices.

Blood pressure

The best thing to do for *high blood pressure* is to go on a juice fast. Juices supply blood and tissues with the important mineral, potassium, which helps to eliminate accumulated sodium chloride (salt) from the tissues. A juice fast for high blood pressure should be of three to four weeks duration. Usually in this period of time the blood pressure goes down to normal. This therapy can be repeated several times with an interval of six months between each fast. The most suitable juices for high blood pressure are citrus fruits, black currants and grapes, plus carrots, spinach, parsley, nettles, onions and garlic (as an addition). Even in *low blood pressure* a juice fast can be tried, preferably under a doctor's supervision. In this case the useful juices are pineapple, celery, nettles, black radish, onion and garlic in addition to carrot, beet and grape juice.

For *edema,* or water-logged body tissues, juices of pears and dandelions are used.

Leg ulcers

Leg ulcers heal faster with raw juice therapy. Juices of onion and garlic are added to carrot juice. Also effective are citrus and apple juices. A dressing of cabbage leaves and yellow onions over the ulcer speeds the healing process.

Obesity

Raw juice fasting is obviously a very appropriate therapy for *obesity*. Juices of celery, watercress and nettles are specifically valuable. The duration of treatment is three to four weeks, or even much longer if necessary. You can read in Chapter 2 of this book how one 59-year-old woman fasted on liquids for 249 days and lost 74 of her 262 pounds.

Rheumatic diseases

Rheumatic diseases are particularly responsive to juice therapy. Fasts of four to six weeks can be recommended. The alkaline action of raw juices dissolves the accumulation of deposits around the joints. The combination of other biological therapies is advisable—massage, hydrotherapies, etc. (see Chapter 9). In cases of *gout*, a noticeable worsening of the condition may develop in the early stages of fasting when uric acid, dissolved by juices, is thrown into the blood stream for elimination. In very advanced cases it is difficult to bring about a permanent improvement, but juice fasting always causes a definite improvement in the condition. Serious *arthritic* deformities cannot be corrected, of course, but the function of the deformed joints can be greatly improved. Juices most valuable in these situations are carrot, beet, and celery. Even juices rich in vitamin C can be used. Rheumatic diseases are collagen diseases and vitamin C is essential for healthy collagen.

Diabetes

Even *diabetics* can try juice therapy, *but only under a sympathetic doctor's control.* The carbohydrate content of juices is not high; besides, a certain amount of carbohydrate is good for diabetics. (Fat is burned in the "fire" of the carbohydrates!) The leg ulcers of diabetics heal faster during juice therapy. Young diabetics should engage in sports; heavy physical work and exertion diminish the need for insulin.

Juices for the treatment of diabetes are: green beans, nettles, cucumber, celery, watercress, lettuce, onions, garlic and citrus juices. Cucumber contains a hormone needed by the cells of the pancreas in order to produce insulin. The hormones contained in onions are also beneficial in diabetes. Note: bean skin tea is considered by many biological doctors to be a natural substitute for insulin and extremely beneficial in diabetes. The skins of the pods of green beans are very rich in silicic acid and certain hormonal substances which are closely related to insulin. One cup of bean skin tea is equal to at least one unit of insulin. The recommended dose: one cup of bean skin tea morning, noon and evening (Waerland).

Kidney disorders

Kidney diseases and *prostate disorders* can be coped with successfully with raw juices. The juices of horse radish (small amount), watercress and birch leaves can be added to carrot and celery juice. Lemon juice is effective in dissolving uric acid stones in the bladder. For prostate disorders, pumpkin juice is reported to be specifically beneficial.

Skin diseases

Various forms of *eczema* and other skin eruptions have been successfully treated for years with fasting methods. A certain worsening of the condition can be expected in the beginning, due to the increased elimination of waste matter. The colorful juices of black currants, red grapes, carrots, beets, spinach, and nettles are recommended. Cucumber juice, internally and externally, is specifically advised for the treatment of skin diseases; it possesses acknowledged cosmetic properties.

Nervousness and insomnia

Recommended juices for conditions of nervousness and insomnia are apples, carrots, oranges and celery.

DO-IT-YOURSELF RAW JUICE TREATMENT

In the limited space of one chapter it would be impossible to give all the facts and answers related to the vast and complicated subject of raw juice therapy. I hope, however, that this presentation will serve as a stimulus to use raw juices, this time-proven biological remedy, in the treatment of many disorders where orthodox medical treatments are helpless.

In the case of serious conditions, such as diabetes, low blood pressure, acute conditions and serious infections, etc., it would be advisable to undertake raw juice therapy under expert professional control.

In chronic and less serious conditions, and particularly when used as a prophylactic measure, raw juice therapy can be safely undertaken on your own. The most effective therapeutic way to use raw juices is in conjunction with fasting. In Chapter 2 you will find detailed instructions on how to go about undertaking do-it-yourself raw juice fasting. Follow the instructions carefully, especially the instructions regarding the breaking of the fast.

In addition to their pure medicinal property in the treatment of practically any disease, raw juices have an extraordinary revitalizing effect on all the vital organs of the body. The miraculous rejuvenating property of a raw juice diet is well known by all beauty farms and rejuvenating clinics, where raw juices are used extensively. The magic beautifying, "youthifying" and rejuvenating effect of raw juices is due to their cleansing and detoxifying property. Raw juices purify the blood and all the tissues of the body, neutralize the waste products of metabolism, and help in building new tissues. They are indeed rightfully called "the internal bath of health and youth."

PRACTICAL POINTS TO REMEMBER

1. All raw juices should be freshly prepared.

2. Use an electric juice extractor. The large department stores and the health food stores carry various types. Follow the instruction booklet that comes with the juicer.

3. Use only fresh vegetables and fruits, preferably organically grown (available at better health food stores and organic farms). If vegetables and fruits are bought from the ordinary supermarket they have probably been heavily sprayed with poisonous insecticides and waxes. Wash them very carefully. I use warm water and soap or a mild detergent to wash such vegetables and fruits as apples, pears, grapes, plums, cucumbers, carrots, green peppers, tomatoes and celery. Rinse well, three or four times, in progressively colder water. Give the final rinse under running water, rubbing vigorously with a brush and with your hands.

4. Make only as much juice as needed. In storage, even in the refrigerator, raw juices rapidly lose their therapeutic and nutritional value.

8

How the Magic Power of Fever and Over-heating Therapies Helps to Restore Health

"Give me a chance to create fever and I will cure any disease," said the great physician Parmenides two thousand years ago.

"High temperature during infection helps combat the growth of virus. Therefore, fever should be not brought down with drugs," said a great modern healer, Nobel prize winner, famous French virologist and professor of medicine, Dr. A. Lwoff.

Why then do mothers get so anxious when Junior suddenly develops a slight fever? They run to the family doctor and with the help of many modern fever-suppressing drugs quickly bring the fever down "to normal."

Fever has been too long a misunderstood and mistreated symptom. Most medical doctors try to combat and suppress fever. They see in fever a negative, pathological condition which must be eliminated as fast as possible. The biological doctor or nature-cure practitioner considers fever to be a constructive, healing-promoting symptom, created by the body in its effort to fight infection or other diseased conditions and restore health.

PHYSIOLOGY OF FEVER

The human body is the most complex and most perfectly designed construction in creation. Its ingeniously designed system has been perfecting itself for thousands of years. Forced to fight rugged conditions of nature and a hostile environment, the body has developed an effective defensive mechanism to meet the "demands of stress." It has, among other things, its own healing capacity which is greater than the medical sciences can ever hope to achieve. The human body is equipped with the most intricate defensive, healing and restorative system capable of facing all kinds of infections, health-abusing practices, and physical and mental stresses which may threaten its health or life. A complex glandular system—particularly the lymphatic glands, tonsils and endocrine glands—forms a defensive line against hostile invaders and other factors which pose a threat to the organism. If this Maginot Line is broken, there are other forces on the second line of defense ready for action. *Fever is one of these second-line defensive and healing forces.*

When the first line of defense is broken and the infection is taking hold, the body initiates a new drastic emergency measure in the form of a raised temperature. The high temperature speeds up metabolism, inhibits the growth of the invading virus or bacteria, and literally burns the enemy with heat. This is not wishful thinking but a scientific fact, proven by Dr. Lwoff in many experiments. Many biological doctors, who use fever as their ally, can testify that fever, indeed, is a "great medicine."

Fever is an effective protective and healing measure not only against cold and simple infections, but against such serious diseases as polio[1] and even cancer.[2] In biological clinics in Europe, overheating therapies have been effectively used also in the treatment of rheumatic diseases, skin disorders, insomnia, and muscular pains.

How malaria prevents and cures cancer

About twenty years ago the great Pontine swamps, not far from Rome, Italy, presented a constant source of malarial infections. Then the swamps were dried out and malaria disappeared. But a remarkably strange observation was made recently. While earlier the whole malaria-infected area was free from cancer, now, twenty years later, the population there shows the same incidence of cancer as the rest of Italy. This shows that the frequent fever attacks, common in malaria patients, stimulated the body's own defenses so that cancer could not develop. This incident was reported by the famous German cancer specialist Medical Professor Werner Zabel.[3]

Too weak to have fever

Those who do not understand the nature and purpose of fever are often puzzled by the fact that some elderly patients do not get fever, even when they are suffering from severe infectious disease. Post-mortem examination may show that they have died of a severe infection, yet their temperature never went up; sometimes it even remained slightly subnormal. The biological doctor, who sees fever as the body's own healing measure, puts the pieces of the puzzle together easily: The patient was too weak and debilitated, and simply didn't have the strength to mobilize the body's defensive forces. He was, in other words, too weak to get fever!

SCHLENZ-BATH FOR INCURABLE DISEASES

Back in 1932, Maria Schlenz, an Austrian lay-woman, wrote a remarkable book, *So Heilt Man Unheilbar Scheinende Krankheiten —So Are Cured Incurable Diseases.* After the second World War her method was scientifically tested and later incorporated into the standard arsenal of therapies in many university hospitals. Now the Schlenz-method of overheating therapy is employed widely in Europe, particularly by the biological clinics. Prof. Werner Zabel, the leading biological doctor in Germany, uses Schlenz-bath in his clinic in Berchtesgaden and testifies that it indeed does cure "incurable" diseases.

Here is how the curative Schlenz-bath is taken:

First, the patient should not eat for at least two hours before treatment. If possible, the bladder and the colon should be emptied. The bath tub should be as large and as deep as possible. Most American type tubs are too small for this treatment. European bath tubs are about twice the size of the average American tub.

The patient must be *totally covered with water,* including his head; only his nose, eyes and mouth—and as little as possible of them—should be left uncovered. Start with a low temperature of about 36° C, or approximately the temperature of the skin. Let warm water run slowly from the faucet and stir constantly. In 15 to 20 minutes bring the temperature in the tub to about 38 or 39 degrees centigrade, later up to 40 and perhaps a little higher, depending on the patient's reaction. The length of the treatment is about one hour. Since the temperature in the Schlenz-bath is not very high (some may remark that they take a tub bath hotter than this), how could this bath possibly have a curative effect? The secret is that if the body is *totally* covered by water there is no heat escape from the body and its temperature will invariably rise to match the temperature of the water.

The Schlenz-bath, if given to sick patients, must be supervised. Pulse should not go over 130 or 140. The temperature of the water should be controlled at all times with a thermometer. If the patient feels any discomfort, he should be raised out of the water to a sitting position for awhile. It is also recommended that the nurse massage the patient with a stiff-bristled brush during the bath. This brings the blood to the surface of the skin and relieves the heart from undue pressure.

STEAM BATH

While modern medical science is in the process of discovering the therapeutic benefits of overheating baths, people in many countries have instinctively and for thousands of years used the same methods on their own for the prevention and healing of sickness. The Romans had their hot baths more than two thousand years ago. The Japanese use very hot baths and claim that they have an invigorating and rejuvenating effect. Russia has over a thousand-year-long tradition of steam baths. The Turkish baths are famous around the world for their dry air and very high temperature. But perhaps the country most famous for steam baths is a little, cold Northern country with rugged and brave people—Finland.

FINNISH SAUNA

In Finland, the steam bath, or *sauna,* is an historic tradition. For over a thousand years the sauna has been an important part of Finnish life and Finnish culture, cherished by every Finnish man, woman and child. The sauna is credited for much of the rugged vitality and endurance—the *sisu*—of the Finnish people.

In a country of less than 5 million people, there are an estimated 700,000 steam bath facilities—one sauna for every 7 people! Most Finnish saunas are in separate buildings specially constructed for this purpose. Every farm has its own sauna, usually built on the shore of a lake or river. Most family houses in the city have saunas built on the lot, usually in the back yard.

Finnish sauna bathing starts with *löyly*, which is the Finnish word for steam. Water is thrown over hot stones, hot steam fills the room and raises the temperature. The bather can sit on a low or high bench, depending on the temperature he prefers. The usual temperature for a Finnish sauna is about 212° F, sometimes even higher. For the uninitiated I would not advise temperatures higher than 180–190° F.

In order to further increase the effect of heat and stimulate sweating, the Finns use birch brooms, *vihta*. Fresh birch branches with leaves are tied together to form a short broom. They are used fresh in summer or dried in winter. The dried broom is dipped in warm water and regains the same shape as the fresh one. Bathers hit themselves all over with these birch brooms. It may seem odd and eccentric to the uninitiated, but you have to try it for yourself to appreciate the fantastic delight and unbelievable pleasure the sauna with a birch broom can give.

After hot *löyly*, bathers usually jump into the nearby lake or river, or in winter they run out and roll in soft snow. What an exhilarating and delightful experience! Then they return to the sauna and warm up again, either by sitting up on the benches or taking more *löyly* with the brooms. Following this they wash themselves with warm water and soap and finish by throwing a bucket of cold water over themselves. In modern saunas, of course, there are showers and even swimming pools.

Finally, the bathers take a long relaxing rest on the benches in the dressing room and allow the wide-open pores to close, perspiration to cease, and the body to return slowly to normal temperature.

Therapeutic properties of sauna

In addition to the prophylactic and therapeutic benefits of an artificially raised fever, which a prolonged steam bath always ac-

complishes, the sauna bath is specifically conducive to profuse therapeutic sweating. Many toxins, accumulated in the system as a result
of metabolic wastes and sluggish elimination, are thrown out of the
body with perspiration. The skin is our largest eliminative organ,
"the third kidney." The skin should eliminate 30 percent of the
body wastes by way of perspiration. Hundreds of thousands of tiny
sweat glands act not only as the regulators of body temperature, but
also as small kidneys, detoxifying organs, ready to cleanse the blood
and free the system from health-threatening poisons. When the
kidneys cannot eliminate the normal quantities of urine due to
overwork or a weakened condition, the body tries to eliminate such
wastes by way of the skin. Uric acid, a normal compound of urine, is
found in large amounts in the perspiration. The chemical analysis of
sweat shows that it has almost the same constituents as urine.

The American conception of the sauna seems to be that it is
helpful in reducing weight by eliminating several pounds of water
through sweating. But the benefits of the sauna are far beyond mere
reducing. You not only lose water by sweating in the sauna, but
sweating also cleans your body of toxins, wastes and impurities.

Thus, the prophylactic value of a steam bath for normally
healthy people wishing to stay healthy and prevent illness, is easy to
realize. However, the therapeutic value of sauna is just as great as the
prophylactic.

The therapeutic property of sauna is attributed to the following
facts:

- Overheating with *löyly* stimulates and speeds up the metabolic
  processes and inhibits the growth of virus or bacteria.
- The vital organs and glands are stimulated to increased activity.
- The body's healing and restorative capacity is accelerated.
- The eliminative, detoxifying and cleansing capacity of the skin
  is dramatically increased by the stimulating action of the sweat
  glands.
- The body is thoroughly cleansed and rejuvenated inside and
  out.

Many authorities attribute the phenomenal therapeutic properties of sauna to the Finnish custom of jumping into cold water or
snow during bathing. The sudden changes in temperature are known
to stimulate adrenal glands; the effect of the alternate hot and cold
bath is likened to a cortisone injection.[4]

DO-IT-YOURSELF SAUNA

If you do not have your own sauna, what can you do and how can you use fever to stimulate and strengthen your own defenses against infections and other diseases?

Here are few things you *can* do:

1. Do not suppress or reduce, but support and sustain fever in colds and acute infections.

2. You can take Schlenz-bath, as I described in this chapter, in your own bathroom. If you plug the emergency outlet with some pieces of cloth or paper, you will be able to raise the water in your tub so that it will cover your whole body—but be careful not to flood your house!

3. Physical activity to the point of heavy perspiration is almost as beneficial, if not more so, than the overheating bath. Physical exertion may actually raise body temperature several degrees. A combination of heavy exercise or exhausting, perspiring games, with swimming in a pool or the ocean can substitute for a Finnish sauna.

4. Even if you don't have a bath tub, a do-it-yourself sauna in your own bedroom can be made as follows: Wrap yourself in a heavy bath sheet. Put a plastic or rubber sheet on your bed to protect it from damage by perspiration. Take one or two hot water bottles and lie on the rubber sheet. Cover yourself with an electric blanket turned on high, leaving just a crack for breathing. Use several heavy blankets if necessary. Remain until profuse sweating occurs—half an hour or more. Finish your do-it-yourself sauna with a cold shower or rub-down.

Warning. Although a fever is a welcome, constructive symptom and is perhaps the best "medicine your body could have," and therefore should not be suppressed or lowered, but supported and sustained, I do not want to leave you with the impression that fever should be simply ignored. Fever is a serious matter, good and beneficial, but serious nevertheless. In small babies particularly the heat-regulating mechanism is not fully developed and a sudden temperature rise may cause convulsions. The sudden rise of temperature in adults to over 103° F should be watched carefully as it may become dangerous, according to some authorities. Some other doctors believe that fevers up to 104° or 106° are not harmful in themselves.[5] It is wise, however, to have an understanding doctor supervise a patient with a high fever and watch for possible dangers in the development of the disease.

THE BIOLOGICAL TREATMENT OF COLDS

The biological doctor would give the following prescription to a patient with a high fever due to a cold or acute infection:

1. Stay in bed and keep warm.
2. Fast; consume no foods at all until the fever is gone.
3. Do not take aspirin or other fever-suppressing drugs.
4. Try to induce the body to perspire by drinking lots of warm drinks. Citrus juices mixed with warm water and sweetened with honey are beneficial.
5. Take large doses of vitamin C. Dr. W. J. McCormick, the world's greatest authority on the therapeutic uses of vitamin C, is reported to recommend massive repeated doses of 500 to 1000 mg. in acute infections. In severe cases the doctor can give vitamin C injections intravenously. Otherwise take vitamin C orally. Doses of 500 or 1000 mg. every hour will rapidly neutralize bacterial or viral toxins in the body and will usually bring down fever within a few hours. This dramatic chemotherapeutic action of vitamin C has been clinically demonstrated in extensive experiments. Vitamin C will accomplish a rapid lowering of fever, not because it will suppress it, but because it will help the body's own defenses to win the battle with the bacteria or virus and thus make the continuation of fever unnecessary.

Note: Vitamin C is non-toxic and completely harmless, even in massive doses.

9

How Arthritis Is Cured in Europe

Arthritis is not only the most agonizing and crippling, but also one of the fastest-growing of all degenerative diseases. There are over thirteen million arthritis sufferers in the United States.

While official medicine admits its inability to penetrate the mysteries of arthritis and find effective treatment for it, biological medicine, a new, fast-growing branch of medical science in Europe, offers a new hope for the sufferers of this agonizing disease. The biological clinics in Europe have developed new methods of treatments which have proven to be most successful in healing many diseases, including arthritis.

I have spent several years in Europe and studied first-hand these biological methods and the results obtained with them. I have visited many clinics in Sweden, Germany and Switzerland. I have interviewed staff physicians in these clinics and talked to hundreds of patients. I have seen with my own eyes how patients with arthritis, crippled for years, have left their crutches and beds and walked.

I have described in detail the full story of successful biological cure for arthritis in my book *There Is a Cure for Arthritis,* published in 1968 by Parker Publishing Company, West Nyack, New York. The Foreword for the book is written by Lars-Erik Essen, M.D., one of the leading pioneers of biological medicine and the director of Vita Nova, the health resort in southern Sweden. Several other medical doctors have collaborated with me on this book. It contains complete do-it-yourself biological therapies for arthritis, the answers to many of the common and pertinent questions the sufferers of arthritis have about diet, climate, vitamin supplements, cortisone, citrus fruits, vinegar, high protein diets, etc., in addition to a large list of actual cases, described in detail. Later in this chapter I will report several such cases taken from Swedish biological clinics.

WHAT IS ARTHRITIS?

There are many different forms of arthritis. The most common types are rheumatoid arthritis and osteoarthritis. Together they are responsible for over 90 percent of all the cases of arthritis.

Osteoarthritis is usually believed to be the result of "wear and tear" on the joints during a long life. It usually affects people past middle age. It is characterized by degenerative processes in the joints, softening and erosion of the cartilage enlargement of the affected joints. The weight-bearing joints are usually affected first, but any joint of the body is vulunerable to osteoarthritis.

The most serious form of arthritis is, however, rheumatoid arthritis. It is an extremely painful and crippling disease which affects people of all ages, but particularly young adults who are in their most active and productive period of life. Women are afflicted with rheumatoid arthritis three time as often as men. Rheumatoid arthritis usually starts with an inflammation of the synovial membrane which eventually leads to deposits in the joints, bone degeneration, deformity, and a subsequent invalidity if proper treatments are not instituted in time.

WHAT CAUSES ARTHRITIS?

It is important to realize that although swollen and inflamed joints may seem to be the very first signals of approaching arthritis, they are not at all the first symptoms of the onset of the disease. *Arthritis is not a local disease of a particular joint but a systemic disorder; a disease which affects the whole body.* It takes years and years of abuse to bring about the systemic disturbance in the bodily functions which eventually leads to a breakdown of the health and the functions of the joints. The arthritic patient usually suffers from a general deterioration of health in the form of sluggishness in the function of his vital organs; incomplete digestion and assimilation of foods; nutritional deficiencies; glandular disorders, particularly in the endocrine system; impaired elimination of metabolic wastes and toxins; and a weakened nervous system and circulation. These systemic disturbances affect the biochemical structure of the various tissues of the body and cause what one of the pioneer practitioners of biological medicine in the United States, R. P. Watterson, M.D., calls a "biochemical suffocation."

In order to understand the nature, causes and mechanics of the development of arthritis, the following basic premises should be kept in mind:

1. Arthritis is not an unrelated, localized disease of certain joints. It is a systemic constitutional disease which always affects the entire body.

2. Arthritis is caused by metabolic disorder and systemic disturbances, particularly in glandular activity, which bring about pathological biochemical changes in all the tissues of the body, specifically in collagen.

3. These biochemical disorders cause inflammatory and degenerative changes in the functions of joints and their surrounding connective tissues.

4. The underlying causes for the development of conditions leading to arthritis are to be sought in prolonged abuse to which the body has been subjected, such as faulty nutritional patterns, overeating, nutritional deficiencies, lack of exercise, unchecked chronic infections, and severe emotional and physical stress. These health-destroying factors eventually result in diminished vitality and lowered resistance to disease, diminished glandular activity and hormonal imbalance, intestinal sluggishness, impaired elimination and autointoxication.

THE PROGRAM OF SUCCESSFUL
BIOLOGICAL TREATMENTS

It is self-evident that the only measures that can be successful in correcting arthritis, bringing it under control and accomplishing a lasting cure, must be ones which are directed at correcting its underlying causes. Prolonged use of drugs, even such "simple" drugs as aspirin, will eventually suppress and break down the body's own defensive and healing mechanisms and cause severe chemical and hormonal imbalance. The disease will then be pushed further and further toward a condition where it will be completely incurable.[1]

Therefore, in order to obtain lasting results the total withdrawal of all drugs is imperative.

Biological treatments are directed at:

1. Eradication and correction of abnormal and health-destroying conditions which have led to the development of the disease.

2. Assisting the body's own healing forces in normalizing all the metabolic processes; establishing biochemical stability; cleansing the body of accumulated toxins and wastes; strengthening the functions of all the vital organs; revitalizing glandular activity and achieving a hormonal balance—or, in sum total, rebuilding and strengthening the general health of the patient.

When the causative factors are thus eliminated and the body is strengthened and revitalized by proper dietetic, physiotherapeutic and other biological measures, *then the organism's own curative powers are given a chance to take over* and bring about the actual cure.

Therapeutic fasting

Almost without exception the treatment of arthritic patients in European biological clinics begins with fasting. Fasting is *the one most important curative measure in the treatment of arthritis.*

In Chapter 2 of this book you will find a complete and detailed description of fasting and how it is done in European biological clinics. I only wish to add here that most clinics employ *repeated juice fasts* for patients with arthritis; for example, one week of fasting followed by one week on a special diet, then a two-week long fast followed by two weeks of dieting, and so on. At the famous Buchinger Clinic in Germany, the usual length of fasting is 14 to 21 days. The longest recommended fast for therapeutic purposes is 40 days.

THE PROGRAM OF FASTING
FOR PATIENTS WITH ARTHRITIS†

Fasting (3 to 40 days)

On the first day of fasting only: one hour before enema, two tablespoons of pure castor oil with a glass of water to which the juice of half a lemon has been added.

---

† As it is directed at Björkagården Institute in Sweden.

7:00 A.M.	Morning beverage: vegetable broth.*
7:10 A.M.	Dry brush massage (see description in Chapter 11).
7:30 A.M.	Massage and hot-and-cold shower.
8:00 A.M.	Enema. (At Björkagården an enema is given three times a day during the entire length of the fasting.)
9:00 A.M.	Glass of carrot juice or diluted fruit juice.
10:00 to 11:00 A.M.	Baths: Kuhne-bath (temperature 12–18° C). Alternating sitz baths (warm, 15 minutes, 38° C; cold, half a minute, 18° C). Sauna bath.
11:00 A.M.	Cup of herb tea.*
12:00 P.M.	Massage, exercises, walks.
1:00 P.M.	Enema.
1:20 P.M.	Glass of carrot juice or vegetable broth.
1:30 to 3:30 P.M.	Rest.
3:30 P.M.	Specialized baths.
5:00 P.M.	Glass of fruit juice.
7:00 P.M.	Cup of herb tea.
8:30 P.M.	Enema.
9:00 P.M.	Bedtime.

DIET BETWEEN FASTS

Note: The use of enemas is continued morning and evening during the dieting period until the natural rhythm of the bowel movements is established.

UPON ARISING:	"Excelsior" drink.*
BREAKFAST:	Fresh ripe fruit available in season, preferably sweet fruit: apples, grapes, berries, pears, peaches, etc. Oranges and grapefruit not more than twice a week. Raw nuts, sunflower seeds, linseed meal, sprouted grains and seeds.
BETWEEN MEALS:	Glass of fresh carrot juice, or carrot and celery juice.
LUNCH:	Potato cereal*
or:	Homemade vegetable soup without salt and spices. Use natural herbs for seasoning. Kelp powder can be used as salt substitute.

DINNER: Large bowl of fresh tossed vegetable salad.
Especially recommended vegetables are: carrots, beets, celery, onions, yellow turnips,
and all leafy green vegetables, such as curly
kale, parsley, lettuce, chives, etc.
Boiled or baked potatoes with jackets.

Note: Dinner and lunch can be interchanged.

Fresh vegetable juices and broths plus herb teas, sweetened with honey, are used between meals and at bedtime.

In addition to the above, arthritis patients receive vitamin supplements C, B₁₂, E, a mineral preparation, kelp and cod liver oil.

When the patient's health has begun to improve, small amounts of whole-grain bread, preferably sour-dough rye bread,* homemade soured milk* and homemade cottage cheese* are added to the diet.

It is the general observation of biological doctors that the diet of arthritis sufferers has been deficient in vital nutritive elements for prolonged periods, and has been loaded with overcooked, canned, devitalized and over-refined foods. This sort of nutritional abuse contributes to the general breakdown of health, diminishes resistance to disease, and triggers the development of the degenerative processes in the joints.

In order to reverse the process, rebuild health and initiate an improvement in the patient's condition, a radical overhaul of his dietary habits is of prime importance. The diet must be as easy as possible for the digestive system to handle and, at the same time, provide all the nutrients required for the repair and building of a healthy body.

The diet between fasts, and during the first two to four weeks after fasting, should consist mainly of raw fruits and vegetables (Frischkost), plus raw nuts, seeds and sprouted grains. Uncooked foods will supply not only all the necessary vitamins and minerals, but also very important enzymes and easily digestible natural starches and proteins, all of which are needed for the healthy functioning of the body. The great advantage of such a diet is that it will cause a minimum of waste retention and sluggishness in the digestive organs and will help the body in its cleansing and detoxicating process. It is a purifying, cleansing, and health-restoring diet.

---

* Wherever they appear, asterisk (*) indicates that the recipe or direction cited may be found in Chapter 16.

DRY BRUSH MASSAGE

Dry brush massage is considered an extremely important therapeutic measure in biological clinics. It stimulates the circulation, brings blood to the skin, keeps skin clean from dead cells and impurities, and opens the pores. The skin is your largest eliminative organ and it is of vital importance that it function efficiently. (See Chapter 11 for instructions.) The best time for dry brush massage is right after a cold shower in the morning and before going to bed.

HOT AND COLD SHOWER

Biological clinics attach great importance to alternating hot and cold showers, particularly for patients with arthritis. These showers are always taken in the morning.

The procedure is as follows: First, a warm shower for about five to ten minutes, to warm up the body. This is followed by a cold shower for half a minute to a minute. The water should be as cold as the patient can stand. Following the shower, the patient receives a vigorous dry brushing with a stiff brush and is rubbed with a coarse towel until he is completely warm.

The importance of the alternating hot and cold shower lies in the fact that it stimulates the adrenal and other endocrine glands and reactivates their functions. Some practitioners call it "a cortisone injection, without cortisone's undesirable side effects."

Therapeutic baths

Therapeutic baths play a very important role in the overall biological therapeutic program. In addition to alternating hot and cold showers, mentioned above, the following baths are employed: whirlpool massage, sitzbath, Kuhne-bath, steam bath, sauna, overheating baths, warm sand baths (Bircher-Benner Clinic), Schlenz-bath, etc. (See Chapters 4 and 8 for detailed instructions on the various forms of baths.)

Herb teas and juices

Herb teas and fresh juices of fruits and vegetables are used both during and after fasting.

The medicinal value of vegetables, plants, and herbs is well known. Herb medicines are the oldest remedy known to man, with the possible exception of fasting.

Better health food stores carry a large assortment of various teas: rose hips, peppermint, milfoil, camomile, etc.

Juices recommended in the treatment of arthritis are: carrot, cabbage, celery, beet, apple, orange, grape, and lemon.

Vegetable broth—a mineral-packed "wonder medicine"

Of particular importance to arthritis sufferers is the healing property of vegetable broth.* It is a highly alkaline, mineral-packed liquid—truly a wonder medicine for arthritis. It combats acidosis, so common in patients with arthritis. Acidosis is a tendency toward a high acidity in the bloodstream and tissues. Vegetable broth helps to normalize the mineral balance in the tissues, which, according to many biological practitioners, is of utmost importance for the effectiveness of the treatment.

Vegetable broth is used extensively in all therapeutic fasting, but for arthritics it is recommended as a standard morning drink (in the form of "Excelsior"*) for continuous use.

Vitamin and mineral supplements

Impaired adrenal function is one of the major characteristics of arthritis. It has been shown in clinical research (by Morgan, Wickson and others) that prolonged deficiency in vitamin C and the two B vitamins, pantothenic acid and B_2, can severely damage the adrenals and result in decreased cortisone production. Vitamin C increases the production and utilization of cortisone.

Therefore, biologically oriented doctors advise heavy doses of vitamin C, 1,500 to 3,000 mg. a day, in the treatment of arthritis. This should be a natural vitamin C, made from rose hips, acerola berries, green peppers, or other natural sources. Natural vitamin C contains, in addition to ascorbic acid, bioflavonoids (vitamin P) — citrin, hesperidin, rutin—which always accompany vitamin C in its natural state, and which make ascorbic acid biologically more effective and potent.

Vitamin B_{12} is also used in the treatment of arthritis with good results. Dosage: 10 to 25 mcg. a day.

Another vitamin useful in treating arthritis is vitamin E. Some researchers suggest that scar tissue, which forms around the joints in arthritis, could develop as a result of vitamin E deficiency.[2] The usually recommended dosage is 300 to 600 I.U. a day.

Minerals are also considered extremely important in the treatment of arthritis. Disturbances in the body's mineral metabolism are usually indicated in arthritis. Therefore, the restoration of proper mineral balance in the tissues is imperative for an effective and fast recovery.

European clinics use various mineral preparations. For the United States, the mineral supplements most useful and easily obtainable would be kelp and bone meal. Recommended doses are reported to be 10 kelp and 10 bone meal tablets a day. Kelp is especially beneficial for arthritis sufferers. It could be used as salt replacement in the seasoning of salads, soups, and other foods. In Japan, where kelp (seaweed) is used extensively as an important part of the daily diet, arthritis is virtually non-existent.

Other supplements

The following food supplements, in addition to the ones mentioned above, are used and recommended by most biologically oriented practitioners:

Brewer's yeast (or food yeast) —about 3 tbsp. a day.
          Note: never use yeast intended for baking!
Cod liver oil, plain, not fortified—1 tsp. a day.
Raw wheat germ—2 to 3 tbsp. a day.
Wheat germ oil—2 tsp. a day.
Lecithin (granules or liquid) —1 tbsp. a day.
Whey, tablets or powder (for better intestinal hygiene) .

In addition, such natural foods as honey, soybeans, sunflower seeds, sesame seeds, raw nuts, yogurt, black molasses, and cold-pressed vegetable oils should be used to make a well balanced and nutritious diet.

Parenthetically, for the best effect and the fullest biological value, all vitamins and minerals and other food supplements should always be taken *with meals.* Because many vitamins are water soluble, and when taken in large doses may be readily lost in urine, it is advisable that the daily dose should be evenly divided between three meals, rather than taken all at one time.

Nutritional taboos for arthritics

It is the opinion of biologically oriented doctors that the best therapeutic diet for arthritics is a low-protein diet, with emphasis on raw, fresh vegetables and fruits, and with the total exclusion of meat and fish. Also, salt, white sugar and white flour and everything made from them, soft drinks, coffee, tea, alcohol, and tobacco should be completely eliminated.

The value of biological treatments for arthritis was scientifically tested by the Royal Free Hospital in London, England, in 1949. Twelve patients with arthritis, all more or less hopeless cases given up by doctors as not responsive to conventional treatments, were selected to participate in the tests, which were carried out under careful scientific control. The experiment was documented on films taken during the entire period of the treatments; both the films and the detailed report were published in the British Medical Journal.[3]

The results were very convincing. Patients who had been considered hopeless cases, crippled and in many cases bedridden, improved remarkably and regained the use of their deformed and formerly immobile joints. They literally left their crutches and beds and walked. The treatments used in this experiment were those employed at the Bircher-Benner Clinic in Zurich, Switzerland—basically a raw food diet and other biological treatments, as described in this chapter.

Biological medicine is not quackery or a passing fad. It is a new, fast growing branch of medical science—truly the medical science of the future. It is as scientific as it is simple. Its philosophy is based on the fundamental principle of intelligent cooperation with nature; it sees man as a part of nature, subject to its eternal laws. It is a modern science which incorporates all the harmless and effective therapies that can be applied in the support of the body's own healing forces in restoring health.

A biological program of treatments is not easy. There are no specific miracle remedies, no specific diets which can cure arthritis. Arthritis can be cured only by the efforts of the body's own healing powers. With the assistance of the wide arsenal of biological treatments (as described in this chapter) and with the full and willing cooperation of the patient, it can be done—it is done in European clinics every day. But in order to achieve lasting and effective results, full cooperation and a positive effort on the part of the patient are imperative.

Lars-Erik Essén, M.D., the leading pioneer of biological medicine in Sweden, said:

> There is no question that arthritis, if not too advanced, can be cured. Biological methods are the only ones at present which can bring about the cure. . . . Many patients have been restored to health through the practiced application of biological medicine after all the conventional treatments have failed. Biological medicine and naturopathic methods of treatment will come to the fore more and more as the successful alternative to conventional therapy; and for the afflicted, who tried in vain conventional therapy, they present the only choice.

Here are a few actual cases of arthritis cures taken from Swedish biological clinics:

CASE HISTORIES

The case of Mrs. Greta Friberg, Eningnäs

This is a true and dramatic story of human suffering and despair, a *circulus vitiosus* of going from doctor to doctor, from hospital to hospital, in the hope of finding relief from agonizing pain. This is a typical story of an arthritic, who consumed astronomical amounts of toxic drugs—and only became worse and worse! Happily, this sad story has a good ending!

The first signs of arthritis appeared in 1964. It started with a certain stiffness in the joints. The stiffness persisted and later the joints became swollen and painful. A visit to a doctor and examination showed low blood values (70 percent) and a high sedimentation rate (65). The doctor sent Greta Friberg to a hospital in Borås.

Thus started a two-year-long history of visits to various doctors and hospitals: two weeks, seven weeks and ten weeks at Boras Hospital, and five weeks at a convalescent home in Hultafors. Her condition was becoming progressively worse, her blood value was only 40 percent and the sedimentation rate 90. Finally after five weeks at the convalescent home, the stiffness and swelling in her joints was somewhat relieved.

But in January 1966 her condition again took a turn for the worse. Not only her joints, but her whole body was swollen. Her doctor told her that the swelling was caused by the drugs she was taking. When she stopped taking the drugs, the pain was so unbearable that she couldn't tolerate it. She felt discouraged and hopeless. Her doctors had tried everything and she was only getting worse. She felt depressed and wanted to die. There was no way out of her inferno of suffering and pain.

At this point some friends told her of Björkagården Institute. Her husband felt that it was worth trying—she could hardly get worse.

She went to Björkagården on March 18, 1966, and was put on a 17-day fast. "It wasn't easy, I must admit. My nerves were bad. I was worried and irritable. But after 17 days of juice fasting, to my surprise, I felt great improvement!" said Mrs. Friberg. The pain was all but gone and her joints regained some mobility.

After one week at home (while the clinic was closed) she returned to Björkagården and was put on a one-week pure-water fast; then she was on a special diet for four weeks. After this she had one more week of fasting. She returned home much improved, but not totally cured.

In June 1966 she returned to the clinic and was put on a 21-day juice fast. "After 17 days I felt that finally my health was returning to me. I could do sit-ups and walk long distances in the surrounding woods," said Mrs. Friberg. It was at this time that I met Mrs. Friberg at Björkagården Clinic and she told me her story.

To complete her cure, Mrs. Friberg returned to the clinic once more on October 9, 1966. This time she stayed a total of eight weeks. There was no more fasting, only a special diet and all the other biological treatments: therapeutic baths, massage, steam baths, etc. Mrs. Friberg returned home completely restored to health. Now she lives a normal life, swims, skiis and exercises regularly. And she continues with the vegetarian diet she learned at Björkagården, which consists mostly of raw fruits and vegetables, cooked potatoes, and little or no bread.

The case of Mrs. Kajsa Andersson, Smålandstenar

After her last baby was born, Mrs. Andersson didn't seem to be able to recover her strength. She was always tired and listless. She could hardly lift her hands. Then came the pain in her arms and hands which led to a visit to a doctor and a dreadful diagnosis—rheumatoid arthritis!

The doctor prescribed drugs and ordered her to stay in bed with warm packs around the affected joints. The warm packs seemed to relieve the pain in the hands, but now it moved to the elbows and the shoulders. Then her legs and feet started to ache. The drugs relieved the pain, but as soon as she was without the pills, the pain returned with increased strength.

After four weeks in bed with increasing disability and pain, which became more and more unbearable, she was sent by her doctor to Spenshults Rheumatic Hospital, one of the most modern medical rheumatic clinics in Sweden. She stayed there six weeks. She didn't receive many treatments except drugs and rest in bed, plus a typical hospital diet, mostly meat, coffee and desserts.

She felt a little better when she returned home, but soon the stiffness and pain reappeared. She was unable to take care of her home and children. She felt discouraged and hopeless.

One day, her nurse brought her a magazine with an article on the Brandal Clinic and biological medicine. After she had finished reading it, she immediately went to the telephone and made a reservation.

She went to Brandal on October 20, 1957. Her condition on arrival was very bad. She could not go up the stairs to her room. She could not dress or undress herself. She was helpless and felt terrible pain with the slightest movement.

The program of treatments at Brandal started with the traditional fast on vegetable broth and carrot juice. Among the other treatments were alternating hot and cold showers, a dry brush massage, and enemas morning and evening. "After one week of fasting I felt so much better that I wanted to continue," said Mrs. Andersson. After the first week she could go up and down the stairs and take short walks outside.

After 20 days of fasting, and one week on a special lacto-vegetarian diet, as described earlier in this chapter, and other biological treatments at Brandal, Mrs. Andersson returned to her home—completely free from her arthritis.

While having a check-up five years later, Mrs. Andersson said, "I am as healthy as anyone could wish to be. I don't remember feeling so well and being so limber and flexible since I was a young girl."

The case of Engineer Karl-Gustav Engberg, Kristinehamn

Mr. Engberg was stricken by disease in 1963. It started with liver trouble and jaundice. He also had suffered from severe constipation for years. Eventually his condition was diagnosed as rheumatoid arthritis.

During the following year he received various treatments from several doctors and hospitals; injections, cortisone, even the so-called injected malaria treatment. Various other remedies were tried without any noticeable improvement. The doctors said that his kind of arthritis was a very rare type that would be difficult to help.

In June, 1964 he went to Björkagården. He could move only with great effort. He was not able to bend his legs or arms. His joints were inflamed, swollen, and stiff.

Mr. Engberg began his treatment with a ten-day fast. He then went on a special diet for 30 days, followed by a new fast for 21 days. He stayed at the clinic for eight months, alternating fasts with diet periods. Some of the shorter fasts were pure water fasts. The long fasts consisted mostly of carrot juice and vegetable broth. The final fast lasted 40 days. The unusually long fasts and the length of his stay at the clinic were motivated by his damaged liver and the necessity of reactivating and rebuilding his liver function as a step in the normalizing of his entire metabolism. All milk was excluded from his diet, but raw nuts and seeds were substituted as a source of protein.

After eight months Mr. K. G. Engberg was able to leave the clinic in perfect health. On returning to his home town, he visited his doctor and received a complete physical checkup. The surprised doctor could not find any traces of arthritis.

Now Mr. Engberg leads a perfectly normal life. He has resumed pathfinding, his favorite sport activity, and he takes part in strenuous training and competitive sports.

The case of Mrs. Ingrid Bengtsson, Borlänge

Mrs. I. B. was stricken with arthritis at the age of 22. She first noticed a swelling in the joints and later stiffness and pain. She was treated with various drugs. Her condition steadily became worse until, in 1958, she had to go to a hospital in Halmstad. She made several hospital visits during 1958–63. In spite of these treatments and the several drugs given her she didn't notice any improvement in her condition.

In 1964 she came to Björkagården Institute. She stayed there three weeks and fasted three times. After three weeks of intensive biological treatments and fasts, her arthritis was completely gone. In answer to my inquiry as to the results of her treatments in Björkagården and the permanency of her cure, Mrs. I. B. wrote, in September, 1966:

"Results were fantastic. No arthritis left . . . No relapses!"

The case of Mr. Martin Lindgren, Borlänge

It started in 1954 with a sore throat followed by tonsillitis. He was treated with various drugs. After awhile he began to have nagging pains, first in his joints and later in his whole body. His doctor in Borlänge diagnosed the condition as rheumatoid arthritis. He had a very high sedimentation rate. The doctor prescribed several drugs, 12 tablets a day, but no cortisone.

In February, 1955, Mr. Lindgren went to Björkagården. He was bedridden with agonizing pains and badly swollen joints.

His first fast, on pure water, lasted ten days, followed by a tenday fast on vegetable and fruit juices. Various baths, massage, vacuum cupping, etc. were included in the program. He fasted a total of 30 days.

After two months in Björkagården Mr. Lindgren was able to return home without the slightest trace of arthritis. During his stay at the clinic he made several visits to his doctor in Borlänge (a nearby city), and each time the doctor reported a steady improvement in his condition, which he attributed to the drugs he prescribed. Mr. Lindgren didn't tell him about his treatments at Björkagården and that he had discontinued the drugs long before. The last examination showed that he was totally free from the disease.

The case has been periodically checked—no relapses in over ten years.

I recently contacted Mr. Lindgren myself to find out if his recovery from arthritis was complete. This is what he wrote to me: "There is nothing wrong with my joints and my general health now. I exercise heavily and feel just great . . . It is tragic that not all arthritis sufferers have knowledge of the methods which restored my health."

10

The European System of Preventing Heart Attacks

Heart disease is the number one killer of Americans. It is reported that well over ten million Americans are afflicted with heart disease. Over 50 percent of all deaths in the United States result from heart disease, which is a much higher percentage than in most other civilized nations. If the term *epidemic* was not limited to infectious diseases, this would be called the most dreadful epidemic in man's history!

The most tragic aspect of heart disease is that many Americans suffer and die from it in the prime of their lives. Men and women in their best years, on the pinnacle of their professional success, just when they should be harvesting the fruits of their labors, succumb to premature death in increased numbers. Recent tests have shown that 70 percent of our young people between the ages of 20 and 25 suffer from various degrees of arteriosclerosis, or hardening of the arteries, which often leads to heart failure.

One of the reasons why we lead the world in heart disease is our failure to develop an effective program of *preventive medicine* in respect to heart disease. Much research money is wasted on trying to find a cure, a drug or a surgical procedure, which will solve the mounting problem of this mass-killer. The plain fact is, however, that the mystery of heart disease was solved long ago. The causes, as well as the means of preventing heart disease, have been known for a long time. Many European countries have used this knowledge to launch massive programs directed at preventing heart disease.

HOW EUROPEAN PREVENTIVE AND RECONDITIONING PROGRAMS SAVE LIVES

The United States has the highest incidence of heart disease of all the civilized countries; Russia has the lowest! The reason is simple: We are looking for a cure—the Russians are concentrating on prevention. The governments of the Soviet Union and other European countries have built over 3,000 rural reconditioning centers where over five million people are treated each year. Tense, fatigued and malnourished workers and executives are given four weeks of reconditioning "treatment," which consists of proper health-building diet, environmental emotional relaxation, and systematic physical training. In addition, they are instructed in rules of good health, proper nutrition and the need for proper exercise, which will guide them when they return to their homes.

Russia also has a nation-wide program of regular physical exercises for everyone, beginning with the schools and continuing with the regular radio-conducted morning calisthenics and exercise breaks in offices and factories.

In West Germany, Switzerland and Austria there are similar preventive programs, financed by governments, insurance companies and private industries. Most heart reconditioning centers are located in the healthy environment of the Alps and the Black Forest of south Germany.

The results of these European preventive programs are there for all to see: the absentee figures among workers visiting these reconditioning centers in Germany have dropped nearly 70 percent in two years;[1] and Russia, as we have seen, has the lowest incidence of heart disease in any civilized country.

WHAT CAUSES HEART DISEASE?

In a nutshell: *faulty nutrition, obesity, smoking, and lack of exercise are responsible for the pathological developments in arteries and abnormal blood-sugar levels which lead to oxygen deficiency in the tissues and eventual heart disease.*

Conversely, wholesome diet, keeping slim, lots of exercise and avoidance of smoking will assure you that you will not be the one of every two Americans who will die from a heart attack.

Of the above-named causes of heart disease, *faulty nutrition is the number one cause.*

HEART DISEASE RELATED TO NUTRITION

At the recent seminar on heart disease in Phoenix, Arizona, the famous heart specialist Dr. Paul Dudley White said that the key to heart disease is in the kitchen. Much heart disease begins in childhood and starts with *overeating.* He blamed mothers for raising a generation of prospective heart cases, and shortening the lives of their children and their husbands, by feeding them too much of the wrong foods. He particularly condemned the starchy foods of the refined carbohydrate category, such as white sugar and white flour, and too much meat, milk and milk products, as the chief fat producers and direct causes of heart troubles.

In order to understand how faulty nutrition can cause heart disease we must understand that health is a harmonious functioning of all the organs of the body, including the arteries and the heart, and is a result of living in a healthy natural environment and eating natural foods. When man's environment and his foods are adulterated—as is the case now with processed, devitalized and poisoned foods, and polluted air and water—then an impairment in the general metabolism of the body results. Nutritional deficiencies, incomplete digestion and assimilation, glandular disturbances, malfunctions of the nervous system, autointoxication, biochemical imbalance in the tissues and blood—all these and many other physiological and degenerative changes are the result of man's adulterated environment and faulty nutrition. Diseases of the heart and blood vessels do not develop suddenly, but rather are the end result of long-time neglect of normal body maintenance.

Faulty nutrition with too much of refined carbohydrates, white sugar and white flour, animal fats, coffee, tobacco, and alcohol, accompanied by lack of exercise, leads to obesity, high blood pressure, hardening of the arteries, digestive disturbances, constipation and many other conditions. Often these may be in so-called sub-clinical stages of which the individual may not be particularly aware. When these pathological changes occur, the body *in self defense* will attempt to cope with the adverse conditions and try to sustain life by adapting to the new situation. When blood vessels become clogged with cholesterol deposits, the heart increases *blood pressure* to assure an adequate blood supply through the narrowed blood vessels. When the digestive and eliminative organs and glands become affected and prematurely wear out or break down, the heart muscle will *enlarge* to cope with the increased amount of work and protect the whole organism from collapse. When the circulation has been so decreased due to the plugged coronary arteries that too little oxygen reaches the heart, pain occurs. This is known as *angina*. Thus, although we have many different forms of heart disease, they are not isolated phenomena but are related to the general health of the body. Heart disease is the result of long-time abuse in the form of poor living habits and faulty nutrition.

HEART DISEASE AND OBESITY

Almost one-third of all Americans are overweight! The Metropolitan Life Insurance Company has found that:

"The death rate is one-third higher among those whose body weight is 20 percent above the average. The death rate from coronary artery disease (heart disease) is 50 percent greater among the overweight."

The well-known American scientist, Dr. C. M. McCays of Cornell University, through his extensive studies has definitely proven that overeating is one of the prime causes of degenerative diseases and premature death; or, as he put it, "the thin rats bury the fat rats."

Overeating

Everyone agrees that the cause of obesity is overeating. But what causes overeating?

Dr. T. L. Cleave, famous British scientist, has a theory which explains what makes us "civilized" people such compulsive eaters. He says that man, like animals, has an inborn instinct which guides him in his choice of the kind and the amount of foods he should eat. He can trust this instinct with absolute confidence, *but only as long as he uses natural substances;* that is, the foods which occur naturally in his environment and are in their natural state. This appetite instinct, however, is "confused" if your food is so over-processed, and so adulterated with artificial flavors and colorings, that it bears very little or no resemblance in either appearance or taste to the original food.

Cholesterol and heart disease

We have been reading and hearing a great deal about animal fats in connection with heart disease. We have been told that the high level of fat consumption, particularly of cholesterol-rich animal fats, is the cause of arteriosclerosis and heart disease.

Now I would be the last person to defend or justify animal fats in human nutrition. But in all fairness it must be stated that it appears as though some scientists are accusing the wrong villain in their attempt to solve the problem of heart disease. Although cholesterol deposits on the walls of the arteries are symptomatic of cardiovascular disease, more and more researchers, particularly in Europe, have become convinced that *cholesterol in itself is not the villain, but that a general biochemical imbalance, impaired metabolism and the resultant inability of the system to handle cholesterol, are to blame!* This view is supported by the fact that many peoples, like Eskimos, some of the North American Indians, inhabitants of Tristan da Cunha, and some tribes in Russian Siberia, consume large quantities of cholesterol-rich foods, yet they do not suffer from hardening of the arteries or heart disease at all. That is, they do not until they adopt "civilized man's" eating habits and start to eat white sugar, white flour, canned foods, and such. There is mounting independent research which shows that cholesterol is an *effect*, not a *cause*.

SUGAR AND HEART DISEASE

Professor John Yudkin of the University of London, England, one of the world's leading nutritionists, has given a hard blow to the theory that the amount of fat in a diet is connected with heart disease. Dr. Yudkin has demonstrated by his studies of two groups of heart patients in a London hospital in 1964 that the excessive consumption of sugar, not of fat, is the prime cause of the epidemic increase of heart disease in civilized countries.[2] Quoting studies made by the Food and Agriculture Organization of the United

Nations, he has shown that sugar consumption has increased in countries with the highest prevalence of heart disease even faster than has fat consumption. In 1966 he and his associates repeated the studies under rigid scientific control and came to the same conclusion: "the person taking a lot of sugar has a greatly increased chance of developing myocardial infarction."[3]

One of the greatest authorities on the sugar vis-a-vis heart topic is M. O. Bruker, M.D., medical director at Eben-Ezers Hospital in Lemgo, Germany. For several decades he has conducted extensive studies on thousands of patients to determine the effect of sugar on their health. He has become convinced that the excessive consumption of white sugar is a major causative factor not only in arteriosclerosis and heart disease, but also in such diseases as caries, digestive disorders, liver and gallbladder diseases, obesity, and even cancer.[4]

Findings of an American physician, Benjamin P. Sandler, M.D., are corroborative to the findings of many European doctors on sugar and heart disease. He also believes that sugar and starches in the diet, not fat, are responsible for the great increase in heart disease. He claims that heart attacks are caused by an *oxygen deficiency in the tissues—which is caused by low blood sugar*—which is caused by overconsumption of sugar and starches. Sounds incredible? Not if you read his book.[5]

How sugar causes heart disease

Here are few proven facts which indict sugar as a causative factor in heart disease:

1. White, factory-produced sugar is an isolated, chemically pure carbohydrate, which can not be normally digested by the digestive organs. All natural foods contain certain nutritive complements—vitamins, enzymes, minerals, trace elements, flavorings, fatty acids, etc.—which are necessary for the effective digestion and assimilation of the nutrients. For example, vitamins E, A, and D cannot be assimilated unless they are accompanied by fatty acids. Conversely, oils cannot be properly utilized without a certain amount of vitamin E. Carbohydrates are not digested or assimilated properly without vitamin B.

2. When sugar in refined form is consumed, the body will use its own storage of B vitamins, particularly B_1, in order to digest it, because sugar is totally void of all vitamins necessary for its digestion. This depletes the body's own supply of B vitamins. Continuous over-

consumption of white sugar can ultimately lead to a B-vitamin deficiency.[6]

3. White sugar also depletes the body of calcium.[7]

4. Overconsumption of sugar and other refined carbohydrates is the major cause of obesity, which is one of the prime causes of heart disease.

5. High carbohydrate intake, especially of refined sugars, causes abnormal fluctuations in the blood sugar level. The heart is a big muscle and its continuous beat is dependent on a steady supply of blood sugar and oxygen. Any interference with the adequate supply of sugar or oxygen to the heart will adversely affect the heart action and may, in serious interference, lead directly to a heart attack.[8] Tests have shown that in more than half of the patients with heart problems there was an evidence of low blood sugar due to high carbohydrate intake.

OXYGEN DEFICIENCY—THE ULTIMATE CAUSE OF HEART DISEASE

There are many contributing causes of heart disease: nutritional deficiencies, overconsumption of sugar and refined carbohydrates, lack of exercise, obesity, smoking, coffee drinking, etc. The way all these factors affect the heart is the same, however: they cause oxygen deficiency in the heart muscle, which, in severe, acute cases, results in a heart attack and death.

The heart is a solid muscle which constantly pumps blood to the billions of cells in the body and it never rests, even for a minute, for the duration of life. It depends in its work on a constant, undiminished supply of fresh oxygen. Even the slightest insufficiency of oxygen supply to the cells of the heart will diminish its efficiency and cause permanent damage. An Austrian scientist, Professor W. Halden, of the World Health Organization, reported to the World Congress for Nutritional Research recently that anemia, for example, may cause degenerative changes in the heart and blood vessels through an insufficient oxygen supply to the tissues by the red blood corpuscles. Tobacco and coffee (also caffeine-containing cola drinks) can also bring about oxygen deficiency by causing violent fluctuations in blood sugar levels and increasing cholesterol and fat content of the blood.[9] Alcohol has a very similar effect.[10] Fatty deposits in the arteries prevent a sufficient flow of oxygen-rich blood to the heart and cause an acute oxygen shortage in the heart muscle.

Thus, in the final analysis, *oxygen deficiency is a direct cause of heart disease.*

VITAMINS AND YOUR HEART

Vitamin E can save your heart

This is where vitamin E enters the heart picture as a miraculous heart saver! Whether it be for an already damaged heart or as a safety measure to prevent an attack, vitamin E is an indispensable aid.

Vitamin E oxygenates the tissues and markedly reduces the need for oxygen. It also has an anti-blood-clotting ability. This anti-coagulant quality of vitamin E prevents deaths through thrombosis or a blood clot. Yet, vitamin E is completely harmless and does not interfere with normal blood clotting in a wound or with the normal healing processes. It has been demonstrated that vitamin E is a dilator of blood vessels, and thus can improve impaired circulation and prevent clots. Vitamin E also prevents production of excessive scar tissue; it even has an ability to melt away unwanted scars. This property is of extreme importance in heart attacks where part of the heart tissue is destroyed.

All of these functions of vitamin E are scientifically confirmed in extensive clinical experiments in many parts of the world. As Evan S. Shute, M.D., of the Shute Foundation of London, Ontario, Canada, the foremost authority on using vitamin E in the treatment of heart disease, says, "Vitamin E is the most valuable ally the cardiologist has yet found in the treatment of heart disease . . . It is the key both to the prevention and treatment of all those conditions in which a lack of blood supply due to thickened or blocked blood vessels or a lack of oxygen is a factor or the whole story of the disease."[11]

It should be self-evident that anyone concerned with the health of the heart should make sure that his diet contains ample amounts of vitamin E. Foods rich in vitamin E are: wheat germ oil, wheat germ, whole grains, unrefined cold-pressed vegetable oils, raw nuts and seeds. But, of course, vitamin E is virtually nonexistent in processed cereals, processed oils, and white flour products. The richest natural source of vitamin E is wheat germ oil—as high as 240 mg. per 100 grams. You can also buy vitamin E in capsule form from your drug or health food store.

Of course, if you have already had a heart attack and are under your doctor's care, it would be advisable not to experiment with any treatment on your own. Show him this chapter and ask his advice on using vitamin E and vitamin E-rich foods. Most doctors who are not too busy to read their professional publications are aware of the benefits of vitamin E. If your doctor is not, it might be advisable to find another doctor; your life may be at stake.

Vitamin C and heart disease

Vitamin C is another vitamin which is seriously involved in heart disease.

The foremost authority on vitamin C in the world, Dr. W. J. McCormick, has shown that the deficiency of vitamin C is one of the causes of coronary thrombosis.[12] Vitamin C deficiency causes ruptures in the blood vessel walls with resultant bleeding which leads to the development of the clot and consequent heart attack. Clinical studies of the vitamin C level in coronary patients showed that 81 percent of them had a subnormal level of vitamin C in their blood.[13]

Russian scientists have found that vitamin C has the ability to drastically lower the amount of cholesterol in the blood. A sharp decline of the cholesterol level—up to 50 percent—was noticed within a 24-hour period after administering ascorbic acid, or vitamin C.[14]

This evidence may suffice to impress upon you that your diet should contain plenty of vitamin C. It strengthens the walls of blood vessels and capillaries, as well as all the connective tissues of the body. It reduces the cholesterol level in the blood and in the walls of the arteries and prevents the development of atherosclerosis and heart attacks. In addition, vitamin C is the most universal of all vitamins in its prophylactic and therapeutic benefits. It is good for your gums, eyes, and skin. It protects against colds and infections, and is an effective anti-toxin. It will protect your body from the harmful effects of many poisons in food and environment and has a protective, buffering action in all conditions of stress. The average American diet is deficient in vitamin C, as has been shown in many studies and tests.

Vitamin B and heart disease

There is much accumulated research which shows that vitamin B also plays an important role in prevention and treatment of atherosclerosis. The B-family vitamins specifically named in this connection are *choline, inositol, pyridoxine, niacin* and *thiamin*.

A study made in Poland on 26 patients with *atheromatosis* showed that 15 of them had a significant decline in blood cholesterol after administration of *niacin*.[15] Another test on 230 patients demonstrated that the death toll of heart patients treated with *choline* was two and a half times smaller than in a corresponding group of patients on conventional medication.[16] And animal tests, conducted at the Washington University School of Medicine, St. Louis, proved that a deficiency of *pyridoxine* (vitamin B₆) has produced in animals the same condition as human hardening of the arteries, as well as high blood pressure. Also *thiamin* deficiency has been found to impair the function of the heart and result in "terminal cardiac standstill."[17]

The best sources of all the vitamins of the B-complex are brewer's yeast, desiccated liver, wheat germ and all the unrefined grains, seeds and nuts. Never use single synthetic B-vitamins, except under a doctor's supervision—some of them could be toxic taken alone in large doses, or they may create a deficiency in vitamins other than the B-complex. B-vitamins are most effective when taken together in natural food supplements, such as brewer's yeast.

Other nutritional factors

Linolenic acid, one of the fatty acids most abundant in linseed oil and soy oil, has been found effective in preventing blood clotting. Norwegian medical researcher, Dr. Paul A. Owren, has demonstrated that one tablespoonful of purified linseed oil a day can prevent heart attacks caused by blood clots. Dr. Owren says that linseed oil is rich in the blood platelet anti-adhesiveness agent known as *linolenic acid*. Most vegetable oils are largely deficient in this fatty acid. Tests with corn or safflower oil, rich in *linoleic acid* (not *linolenic*) showed that they had little or no effect.[18]

Deficiencies in minerals and trace elements have also been shown to play an important role in heart disease. A significant decrease in heart disease mortality could be achieved by an increased dietary intake of *calcium,* reported several researchers in a British medical journal. Other studies have shown that the geographical incidence of cardiovascular disease is higher in soft water areas and lower in hard water areas. Hard water is rich in minerals, including *calcium* and *magnesium,* and trace elements.

A new concept of heart attack has been advanced by a Canadian doctor, P. Prioreschi. On the basis of many experiments from all over the world, he concluded that myocardial infarction is not due to coronary thrombosis, but rather to a metabolic derangement in the tissue. He cites specifically a mineral imbalance as a major contributing cause of heart disease. He names *sodium chloride* (common table salt) as one of the most dangerous cardio-toxic agents. *Potassium* has been found capable of counteracting the heart-damaging effect of cardio-toxic agents and thus preventing heart attacks. A diet containing large quantities of *raw fruits and vegetables* will provide an adequate dietary intake of potassium.[19]

Deficiency in another nutritive element, *lecithin,* is indicated in heart disease. Lecithin is a fatty substance, mostly abundant in soybeans. It has an emulsifying effect on fats, including cholesterol. It has been demonstrated in numerous tests that persons who suffer from coronary thrombosis almost always have a low blood lecithin level. Lecithin prevents clot formation, and thus diminishes the risk of a heart attack.[20] Lecithin supplement to the diets of those who are heavy meat eaters should be of a special importance. Meats are the main sources of cholesterol.

A NINE-POINT PROGRAM FOR A BETTER HEART

The best possible way of solving the growing heart disease problem in the United States would be to follow the European example of a preventive program with a massive network of cardiac reconditioning centers where prospective heart cases could go to rebuild their health and strengthen their hearts. While waiting for action in this direction from our government, life insurance companies, or private industries, here is a 9-point do-it-yourself program for a better heart which can help you to prevent a potential heart attack, or give your already damaged heart the break it deserves.

1. Vital nutrition

See that your diet contains the complete vital nutrition needed to keep your body and your heart in perfect health. An abundance of fresh raw vegetables and fruits, whole grains, nuts, seeds, and beans, with the addition of raw, unpasteurized milk and natural cheese, preferably in the form of homemade fresh cottage cheese,* will supply you with all the necessary vitamins, minerals, complex carbo-hydrates, trace elements, proteins and enzymes needed to build, repair, replace or renew the worn-out cells of your heart, keep your blood well oxygenated and its circulation smooth and strong, and your blood vessels elastic and free from deposits.

2. Food supplements

Supplement your diet with vitamins E, B and C. Use wheat germ oil and vitamin E capsules for vitamin E. Take up to 300 I.U. a day as a preventive dose, and up to 600 I.U. as a therapeutic dose—ask your doctor for the most desirable dosage in your case.

For B-vitamins, use brewer's yeast. Use the dosage suggested on the container, or take three to four tablespoons daily. Or take high potency B-vitamin tablets, made from yeast.

Take rose hips or rose hip tablets for vitamin C—500 to 1000 mg. per day.

In addition to vitamins, use *cold-pressed* vegetable oils, espe-cially linseed or soy oil, for the unsaturated fatty acids (not the usual supermarket type). Dosage: 1 or 2 tablespoons per day. For minerals, especially calcium and magnesium, and trace elements, use dolomite and bone meal tablets, and kelp—all obtained in health food stores. Take 1 tablespoon of lecithin granules each day. Lecithin will not only help in fat metabolism and the prevention of cholesterol de-posits, but is essential for your nervous system and the stimulation of glandular activity.

3. Low animal protein

Excessive amounts of protein, especially animal protein, may harm your heart and your health generally. A study of blood vessel and heart disease in Negroes in St. Louis and in Uganda demon-strates that low-protein vegetarian diet can prevent 90 percent of thrombo-embolic disease and 97 percent of coronary occlusions.[21] A recent study shows that Seventh-Day Adventists, who do not eat meat for religious reasons, have 40 percent less blood vessel and heart disease as compared with the general American public. Dr. Richard Walden, who directed the study, is convinced that the meatless, low-animal-protein diet of these people has much to do with it.

Avoid an excess of meat, especially fat meat in your diet. Do not worry about getting enough proteins. Almost all natural foods con-tain some protein, so, unless you are starving, it is virtually impossible to get too little. The official recommendations for protein requirement are far too high. (See Chapter 6.) A low animal protein diet will help prevent heart troubles; and, when the heart is already affected, will help to restore it to health. A lacto-vegetarian diet of fruits and vegetables with whole grain bread and cereals, beans, sunflower seeds, raw nuts and milk products will supply you with all the proteins you need.

4. Eliminate from your diet:

Sugar in every form: soft drinks, ice cream, cakes, candies, cookies, pastries, jams, chocolate, puddings, syrups, etc. Natural honey can be used for sweetening. Eliminate white flour and white bread and all processed cereals and canned and frozen foods.

Reduce salt intake drastically or cut it out entirely. If absolutely necessary, use sea salt moderately.

5. Keep your weight down

Do not overeat! Every extra inch on your waist, every excess pound you carry around, makes your heart work harder and wears it out sooner. *Remember:* the death rate from heart disease in 50 percent higher among the overweight!

6. Avoid smoking tobacco

A recent survey shows that the death rate from heart disease among women smokers is twice as high as it is for non-smokers. Smoking destroys vitamin C in the body (25 mg. for every cigarette) and causes vitamin B deficiency. It causes constriction of the blood vessels and raises the blood pressure. Smoking disturbs the fat metabolism, raises the fat level of the blood and causes oxygen deficiency, thus contributing to the development of heart disease.

7. Avoid drinking coffee, tea or cola drinks

Coffee, tea, and soft drinks containing caffeine are to the heart what a whip is to the horse. They stimulate and increase the sugar level of the blood temporarily, then drop it down to dangerous levels and cause an oxygen deficiency in heart muscle tissues. Coffee also interferes with iron absorption and may cause a deficiency of inositol, one of the B-vitamins necessary for effective heart function. A good friend of mine was practically living on coffee—10 to 15 cups a day from early morning to late at night. He was constantly boasting that he had never been sick a day in his life, but he dropped dead of a heart attack at the age of 49. Cola drinks, by the way, contain even more caffeine than does coffee.

Warning: If you are a heart case and a coffee addict, be careful how you cut out coffee drinking. Reduce the number of cups per day gradually to condition your heart and avoid distressing withdrawal symptoms.

8. Exercise

There are piles of evidence that the lack of exercise and physical exertion is a major factor in the increasing incidence of heart disease. A British study showed that mortality from heart disease among those who do heavy physical work was less than half that of the group who did little or no physical work.

As I have stated before, the ultimate cause of heart attack is an oxygen deficiency. Outdoor sports, exercise and physical exertion promote the oxygenation of all the tissues of the body, including the heart, increase the blood supply to the heart and strengthen the blood vessels and the muscle tissues of the heart.

Points of warning for heart cases:
- Exercise with caution, prudence and moderation.
- Avoid competitive sports and games.

Walking, up to ten miles a day, is the best form of exercise for the prevention of heart disease.

9. Avoid emotional stress

Fear, greed, hatred, disappointment, insecurity, jealousy, depression, resentment, anxiety, worries, tension, emotional upsets—any or all of these can destroy your heart. According to famous stress-doctor Hans Selye, M.D., all the above mentioned emotional stresses can cause arteriosclerotic lesions. Severe emotional stress causes depletion of vitamin C in the adrenal gland and increases the body requirement for vitamin C—another predisposing factor of heart disease.

"Americans are the most worried people in the world," says Dr. Joshua Bieres, British editor of the International Journal of Social Psychiatry. The highly competitive business climate of the United States is geared to an atmosphere of continuous worry, anxiety and desperation. A typical American businessman or executive does not really know what the terms leisure, relaxation, or a health-building vacation mean. His ultimate in relaxation is a round of golf on a smog-filled city course, where he is trying to close another business deal with his partner! No wonder he worries himself to death at 40 or 50 and leaves a rich widow.

It is my conviction that if you apply the above nine-point do-it-yourself program, you will be rewarded with a better heart which will give you long and friction-free service.

11

How to Help Lower
Your High Blood Pressure—
Without Drugs

High blood pressure—hypertension—is one of the modern diseases which is increasing at an alarming rate. Although high blood pressure is not a real disease, which cripples you or puts you in a hospital, it should not be ignored or dismissed lightly. Many fatalities from cerebral hemorrhage, or stroke, heart attacks or kidney disease are directly linked to high blood pressure. It is estimated that one in every 20 adults, or about six million people in the United States have high blood pressure and that nine million more are in the early stages of it.

WHAT IS HIGH BLOOD PRESSURE?

Your body is crisscrossed by a great network of blood vessels. Through these vessels your heart pumps fresh, clean blood to all the parts of your body to supply all the cells and vital organs and glands with the nutrients they need. Then the blood is returned with the end products of metabolism—wastes and toxins—to be purified by the lungs, liver and kidneys. In order to keep this flow of blood continuous through the relatively narrow blood vessels and make it reach the distant parts of the body, the heart must pump hard and constantly maintain a certain pressure.

This blood pressure can be measured by an instrument called a *sphygmomanometer*. The average, or "normal," *systolic* pressure of adults in good health is about 120 to 130 mm. The *diastolic* pressure is 30 to 40 points lower. The systolic pressure is recorded when the heart is in action; the diastolic when the heart is at rest. It is the higher pressure, or the systolic pressure, that is usually quoted in reference to high blood pressure, although the lower, or diastolic pressure is also important.

There is a wide disagreement among authorities as to what "normal" pressure should be. Most medical doctors, it appears, maintain that 100-plus-half-your-age is normal, which means that as you get older your pressure would automatically increase, so that at the age of sixty the systolic blood pressure of 130 mm would be considered generally normal.

Biologically-oriented medical doctors and naturopathic practitioners have a different view on this. They feel that although it is common for blood pressure to rise with age, it is not a "normal" condition, but a sign that the health of the individual is out of order. The blood vessels may have lost some of their elasticity or they may be plugged with flow-hindering deposits. Or the patient may be suffering from any one of several conditions of disease, which require an elevated blood pressure as the body's own defensive measure. If a person remains in good health and his blood vessels are kept pliable and resilient, he can expect to have a young man's pressure even when he grows older.

A good example of this was Dr. Harvey Kellogg, of the famous Battle Creek Sanatorium. At the age of 72 he had a blood pressure of 118/80—a young man's pressure.

What causes high blood pressure?

Keep in mind that high blood pressure is not a disease, but rather a symptom of other disorders in the body. Hypertension can be due to nervous tension, kidney disease, glandular disorders, obesity, hardening of arteries, etc. In general, it could be said that a great number of diseased conditions in the body will raise the blood pressure. However, by far the most common cause of high blood pressure is the hardening of the arteries. When arteries and arterioles become constricted by cholesterol or other deposits, they lose their elasticity and become brittle and hard, so the blood has difficulty passing through them and the heart has to work harder and increase its pressure in order to maintain circulation. In case of infections or other diseased conditions in various parts of the body, blood pressure is increased as a defensive measure in order to increase the flow of blood to the diseased area, to supply it with the nutrients, hormones and other vital substances needed for the healing processes, to accelerate the detoxification of the blood, and to speed recovery.

BIOLOGICAL TREATMENT OF HIGH BLOOD PRESSURE

As you can clearly see from the above, the objective of the doctor treating high blood pressure should not be to lower the pressure with drugs, but rather to find the underlying causes of the elevated pressure and try to eliminate them. When the underlying causes or diseased conditions are corrected, then the high blood pressure will disappear of itself.

To reduce high blood pressure with the help of drugs is just as unwise as to suppress and combat high fever with drugs. Both are highly beneficial symptoms, initiated and brought about by the body for a defensive purpose: to effectively cope with the adverse diseased conditions and to restore health. Attention should be directed at the real causes of high blood pressure. General toxemia, impaired kidney function, glandular disturbances, hardening of the arteries—these must be corrected.

The biological doctor is concerned not only with the dropping of the systolic pressure, but with the all-round lessening of the strain on the arterial system and the improvement of the general health of the patient. This is accomplished with various biological treatments which are centered around fasting and dietetic restrictions.

HIGH BLOOD PRESSURE AND FASTING

Fasting is considered by most biological medical doctors as the fastest and the most effective therapeutic method of remedying high blood pressure. At the Buchinger Clinic in Bad Pyrmont, Dr. Otto Buchinger stated that high blood pressure is the one ailment for which fasting practically never fails to bring about a complete cure.

He stressed, however, that tobacco is highly injurious to the patient with high blood pressure and advised a total abstinence from smoking.

In Swedish biological clinics practitioners have had the same experience. Ebba Waerland has supervised hundreds of fast cures and reports that high blood pressure is "cured automatically" through fasting and Waerland dietetic therapy.

A case history of lowered blood pressure

Here is one case from Sweden. Mrs. E. P., 44, suffered from high blood pressure for 15 years. In spite of various medical treatments, her pressure continued to climb, and in 1966 it was up to 240. She started her biological treatments in July, 1966, with a ten-day fast on the alkaline juices of fruits and vegetables and vegetable broth.* While fasting she was given an enema morning and evening, plus colonic irrigation twice a week. After ten days of fasting, she was given a salt-free diet of fresh fruits for breakfast, and raw vegetable salad with homemade soured milk and boiled potatoes for lunch and dinner. Bread, butter and cheese were not allowed, except small amounts of fresh homemade cottage cheese.* After two weeks on this diet she was again put on juice fasting for ten more days. I met Mrs. E. P. on the ninth day of the second fast. Her blood pressure had been checked the day before and was down to 137. It had been at that level a whole week. She told me that she felt great, and planned to leave the clinic and go home the following week. She enjoyed her new lacto-vegetarian diet and planned to continue with it at home.

Also in the United States many clinics and nature-cure practitioners have employed fasting very successfully in the treatment of high blood pressure. At Pawling Health Manor, in New York, Dr. R. Cross reported 54 high blood pressure cases treated by fasts between 1957 and 1963. Of these, 38 cases recovered completely and 16 improved.[1] Dr. James McEachen, of Escondido, California, has supervised 141 fasts on patients with high blood pressure at his sanatorium, and reported that all 141 cases were remedied or improved— also a 100 percent result. Similar results are reported from Herbert M. Shelton's Clinic in Texas and Dr. W. L. Esser's Clinic in Florida. Dr. Shelton reported one case in which three weeks of fasting dropped the systolic pressure from 295 to 115.[2]

The general opinion of all practitioners who employ fasting in the treatment of high blood pressure, is that patients who do not respond to the customary treatments, do respond to fasting. Moreover, the cures accomplished by fasting tend to be lasting—provided that good nutritional habits are maintained after the fast.

Points to remember in regard to fasting

1. Although fasting is one of the safest and most practical therapeutic agents known, the general public is largely ignorant as to how it is administered. As with the other therapeutic agents, it is of great importance that fasting be carried out correctly. Misuse or disregard for certain fundamental rules of fasting may make it not only useless, but even harmful. For this reason, before you undertake a fast *make a detailed study of all the facts and advice presented in this chapter and in Chapter 2 of this book.* Of course, I earnestly advise that you discuss your case with an experienced doctor or a nature-cure practitioner, who has had experience with fasts, and, if possible, undertake your fast under his direction and supervision. This particularly applies to cases of extremely high blood pressure, especially if it is accompanied by a weak heart, or if the patient has a record of heart attacks.

2. Two different therapeutic fasting methods for high blood pressure can be considered. One is a traditional water fast, or a complete fast with nothing consumed but water. This is the kind of fast usually employed in American clinics. The other is a fast where the juices of raw fruits and vegetables, plus vegetable broth, are added to the water. The latter is now widely used in most European clinics, and I recommend this method, especially if you fast on your own, without professional supervision. The duration of the fast should be seven to 14 days, depending on the condition of the patient, or how high the blood pressure is.

3. Follow very carefully the instructions given in Chapter 2 on *how to break fast.* This is extremely important. Follow the instructions meticulously.

4. In case of a heart condition or damaged kidney, water drinking should be restricted to a minimum.

5. The mental attitude while fasting is of tremendous importance. The difference between therapeutic fasting and starvation is that while starvation is a negative, undesired condition, accompanied by fear and anxiety, which exerts a negative, disease-producing effect

on bodily functions, therapeutic fasting is a positive, voluntary condition, accompanied by complete confidence and faith in its beneficial effect and anticipated good results. Such a positive attitude stimulates and encourages all the cleansing and healing processes of the body. Therefore, before you start fasting, be thoroughly convinced of its wonderful, beneficial properties. This is also one of the reasons why it is advisable to fast in a clinic surrounded by other fasting patients who can encourage and inspire each other, or under the supervision of a practitioner who can encourage and explain the various symptoms and reactions which may develop during the fast.

HIGH BLOOD PRESSURE AND DIET

If you fast for ten to 14 days in accordance with instructions given in Chapter 2, your blood pressure will probably drop to normal in that period. After the fast is completed it is of great importance to adopt intelligent eating habits, if you wish to prevent the recurrence of high blood pressure.

Your diet should be a *high natural carbohydrate—low animal protein diet,* rich in fresh, raw vegetables and fruits, whole grain bread and unprocessed, whole-grain cereals, nuts and seeds, and low in animal fats. Milk consumption should be cut down, too, but moderate use of yogurt and homemade cottage cheese is allowed. All salt, coffee, alcohol, white sugar, white bread, sweets, strong spices, mustard, and cola and soda drinks, should be eliminated. Also, cut out all refined and processed foods and all fried and greasy foods. A British doctor, Bertrand P. Allinson, who has had wide experience in the treatment of high blood pressure, said the following in regard to the lacto-vegetarian diet suggested above: "My conclusions, based upon a large series of cases, are that dietetic treatment of the lacto-vegetarian type (with not too much stress on the lacto) relieves symptoms in most cases of high blood pressure, reduces the blood pressure in a large proportion of these and keeps the development of fatal complications in abeyance for a long while."

Avoid overeating; keep slim. Eat small meals; chew well. At least once a month fast a few days on fruits or juices. Better still—have a fruit day each week. This will give your heart the rest it deserves.

Food supplements

Supplement your diet with the following food supplements and vitamins which have been found to be of particular benefit in cases of high blood pressure:

1. *Choline.* It has been demonstrated that deficiency in choline, one of the B-vitamins, plays a role in the development of high blood pressure. Patients with dangerous hypertension improved markedly after they had been given choline daily. Their blood pressure dropped and their capillaries were strengthened.[3] Lecithin, made from soybeans, is an excellent source of choline. Brewer's yeast is also an excellent source of choline and all the other B-vitamins.

2. *Vitamin E.* Because vitamin E helps oxygenate the blood and decreases the need for oxygen, it is of special importance for patients with high blood pressure. Vitamin E also dilates the arteries. Wheat germ oil is the richest source of natural vitamin E.

3. *Vitamin C.* Natural vitamin C strengthens the blood vessels and blood capillaries and makes them more elastic. Therefore, more vitamin C in the diet may prevent cerebral hemorrhage caused by weak blood capillaries. It is important to take only natural vitamin C, which also contains vitamin P, or bioflavonoids. Bioflavonoids are of particular importance for the health of blood capillaries. The study made in Russia by Dr. D. E. Dzheims-Levi shows that bioflavonoids, or vitamin P, have a curative effect on high blood pressure. "On the basis of our observations we concluded that vitamin P has a beneficial effect on the well-being of patients and considerably lowers the blood pressure of patients with hypertension—blood pressure rises again when the patients discontinue vitamin P treatment."[4]

4. *Potassium.* It has been demonstrated in animal tests that potassium deficiency can be one of the causes of high blood pressure. It is known that excessive salt intake will cause the loss of potassium. The incidence of hypertension is greater in countries with excessive salt intake. Also, the wide use of refined foods and too few green leafy vegetables in the diet contributes to the very common potassium deficiency. The best sources of potassium are fresh or cooked green leafy vegetables. Avoid salt if you have high blood pressure. Substitute salt with kelp, which is also very rich in potassium.

5. *Garlic.* There is much material in medical literature which suggests that garlic has a dilating effect on blood vessels and is effective in reducing blood pressure. Dr. F. G. Piotrowski, of the Uni-

versity of Geneva, used garlic on 100 patients with abnormal blood pressure, with excellent results.[5]

HIGH BLOOD PRESSURE AND EXERCISE

Strenuous exercises, such as weight lifting and competitive sports, are not advised for sufferers of high blood pressure. They may do more harm than good. But this does not mean that you should resign yourself to a sedentary existence and lie in bed. Quite to the contrary! You should exercise as much as possible. And the best form of exercise for a patient with high blood pressure or heart disease is *walking* accompanied by deep breathing.

Start on level ground and walk slowly for half an hour. Develop a regular breathing pattern. For example, inhale deeply during four steps and exhale during the next six steps. Do this for two to three minutes. After five or ten minutes, repeat the deep breathing again. Breathe as deeply as you can so that all parts of your lungs will be filled with life-giving oxygen-rich air. Also, see that the lungs are completely emptied every time you exhale.

Gradually increase your walking distance each day. If you feel fatigued, take a short rest. Gradually you will be able to walk over a steep landscape without difficulty and increase the duration of your walks up to two or three hours a day.

These walks and breathing exercises will be of great help in lowering your high blood pressure and strengthening your heart. They will stimulate and improve blood circulation, increase the capacity of your lungs, accelerate the general metabolism and increase the elimination of toxins and wastes from your system. All this will have a very favorable effect on reducing blood pressure.

DRY BRUSH MASSAGE

The effective elimination of metabolic toxins and wastes from the system is a prerequisite for the successful treatment of high blood pressure.

The skin is one of the most effective eliminative organs and is, indeed, your largest organ. It is estimated that one-third of body impurities are excreted through the skin. If this organ becomes inactive and its pores choked with millions of dead cells, the impurities will remain in the body and may cause autointoxication and other disorders, including high blood pressure. Inactive skin definitely aggravates high blood pressure.

There are many ways to regenerate your skin activity and increase its eliminating capacity. Heavy physical work will induce perspiration, and hot baths are also excellent. However, in the case of high blood pressure, they are definitely not recommended. The best way to stimulate the skin of the high-blood-pressure patient is to use dry brush massage.

Buy a good natural bristle brush. A coarse bath glove of twisted horsehair or a plant fibre brush could be also used. Do not use nylon brushes; they are too sharp and may damage the skin.

Starting with your scalp, brush vigorously, making circular motions, and massage every part of your body: legs, arms, abdomen, back, etc. Change hands to reach everywhere. Get a brush with an extended handle so you can reach all over your back, too. Brush until your skin becomes rosy, warm, and glowing—about five to ten minutes, or more. Upon arising in the morning and again before going to bed are the best times for massage.

Dry brush massage will benefit you in many ways:
- It will stimulate and help blood circulation.
- It will remove dead skin cells and keep pores open.
- It will help in the elimination of toxins through the skin.
- It will stimulate the hormone- and oil-producing glands.
- It will contribute to healthier muscle tone and better distribution of fat deposits.

All these benefits will be helpful in actuating a reduction of high blood pressure.

After brush massage it is advisable to take a cold shower or a rubdown with a sponge to wash away all dead skin particles from the body.

EMOTIONAL ORIGIN OF HIGH BLOOD PRESSURE

High blood pressure is often called "executive's disease." The overburdened, high-pressured executives of our competitive society become easy prey for high blood pressure, circulatory crisis, angina pectoris, "nervous breakdown," and heart attack.

Stress in the form of continuous worry, psychic pressure, fear, emotional strain, constant tension, combined with regular pick-meups in the form of coffee, cokes, cigarettes, and cocktails, will eventually throw the whole system off balance, physically and emotionally. A devitalized diet of over-processed foods adds to the total picture of constant stress. Insomnia, discontentment, restlessness, weak concentration, headaches, chronic fatigue and irritability will be the first symptoms, eventually followed by high blood pressure and cardiac failure. Nature strikes back in revenge for the violation of the basic biological laws. The body raises the blood pressure to cope with the adverse condition of physical and emotional stress.

It has been clinically demonstrated that any form of stress can increase blood pressure. Anger and fear, smoking, many modern drugs such as cortisone and ACTH, even some vitamins (vitamin E) can raise blood pressure. Unexpressed negative emotions or suppressed hostile feelings can cause blood pressure to go up.

It is self-evident that the underlying causes of emotional origin must be corrected before high blood pressure can be treated successfully. Often, a long holiday "away from it all," free from responsibilities and business pressures, will do more than any drug in the world. This is why European Spas, mineral baths, and reconditioning centers are so effective in restoring the health of tired and overstressed executives.

If the biological treatments outlined in this chapter are not successful, it would be wise to look for possible emotional causes of high blood pressure and eliminate them in order to achieve a complete recovery.

SUMMARY

The successful biological program for bringing blood pressure down and keeping it low must include the following proven measures:

1. Repeated 7- to 14-day *fasts* on fruit and vegetable juices, plus vegetable broth. (See Chapter 2)

2. *Lacto-vegetarian diet,* high in natural raw fruits and vegetables and low in animal protein.

3. Continuous practice of *undereating* and keeping slim.

4. Exclusion of *salt, coffee,* and *alcohol.*

5. Exclusion of *white sugar, white bread* and all *refined* and *denatured foods.*

6. Inclusion of special food supplements:
   - *Vitamin E*—take one to two tablespoons of wheat germ oil each day. Add raw wheat germ to your diet. Take vitamin E capsules, 300 to 600 International Units a day. Note: because vitamin E increases the strength of the heart beat, it may sometimes elevate the blood pressure temporarily. In case of severe hypertension, start with 100 I.U. and gradually increase to 600 I.U. a day.[6]
   - *Vitamin C*—take rose hips in powder or tablet form, or other natural vitamin C supplements, amounting to 1,000 to 1,500 mg. of C a day, and 20 to 100 mg. of rutin or mixed bioflavonoids.
   - *Choline*—take 2 tbsp. of lecithin each day. Supplement your diet with brewer's yeast, rich in B-vitamin complex.
   - *Potassium*—eat lots of green leafy vegetables, potatoes (boiled or baked in their jackets), and other vegetables. Avoid salt. You may also wish to discuss with your doctor the advisability of supplementing your diet with potassium salts in tablet form.
   - *Garlic*—take odor-free garlic and parsley tablets before each meal.
7. Regular walking and deep breathing exercises.
8. Dry brush massage morning and evening.
9. Elimination of possible emotional causes of disease.

The biological clinics in Europe and in the United States have records of thousands of cases of high blood pressure completely cured by the application of the treatments as outlined in this chapter. These treatments are safe and harmless and can be applied by yourself in your own home, if your blood pressure is not too high. In cases of severe hypertension it may be wise to show this chapter to your doctor and ask him about the advisability of undertaking this program of treatment under his supervision.

12

Good News for
Victims of Multiple Sclerosis

Multiple sclerosis is an organic nerve disease, generally referred to as MS. It attacks the whole nervous system, affecting the fatty sheaths which cover the nerve fibres. Since the nervous system regulates all the body's functions, multiple sclerosis brings havoc to the whole organism and affects all the vital organs. It usually starts inconspicuously, with a certain weakness and numbness in the limbs, disturbance in the sense of balance, and dizziness. As disease progresses, the walk becomes more unsteady, the mind becomes affected and emotional changes occur. Often the vision also becomes impaired. Gradually, the disease spreads to the brain, bone marrow, and other vital organs, with increased paralysis throughout the body. Death occurs usually when the lungs and heart muscles become affected.

WHAT CAUSES MS?

Multiple sclerosis is most prevalent in the so-called highly civilized (read: chemicalized!) countries. It is rarely encountered in Italy and the South American countries. Italians and South Americans living in the United States and eating the American diet show, however, the same incidence of the disease as other Americans. Researchers feel, therefore, that there must be a relationship between diet and the incidence of multiple sclerosis.[1] Some surveys in Europe show that the disease seems to increase in areas with a higher consumption of animal fat and milk.[2] Diets low in fat were tried on patients at McGill University in Montreal, Canada, with encouraging results.[3]

In England it was observed that there was an unusually high incidence of the disease in lead-mining areas, which prompted many investigations. It was also shown that the lead content of the teeth of patients with multiple sclerosis was "significantly" higher than that of the control groups.

Many other researchers have linked lead poisoning to multiple sclerosis. The Finnish researcher, Martti Salmi, believes that the incidence of multiple sclerosis is closely related to the occurrence of lead in the soil and the environment.[4] It seems that there is a higher incidence of the disease in the northern hemisphere, with the number of cases increasing as one goes farther north. It has been shown that glacial ice distributed lead-bearing materials to the soils in the northern countries. Also, lead in the air from leaded gasoline is suspected as the cause of the disease.

DIET AND MS

Most research on the relationship between nutrition and multiple sclerosis has been done in Germany. All the accumulated evidence seems to indicate that this crippling disease is caused by malnutrition and is a result of the "civilized" way of life. Researchers have found that the so-called "primitive" people, for example Eskimos and some tribes in Africa and Central America, do not contract multiple sclerosis. However, as soon as Eskimos come into contact with civilization and start to eat white man's devitalized and processed foods, they contract the disease in the same proportion as civilized man. Thus, there is a firm conviction among some investigators that multiple sclerosis is a degenerative disease, caused by nutritional deficiencies and metabolic disorders due to an unnatural, unbalanced diet of devitalized foods. Consequently, all experimental treatments in Europe are centering around a nutritional approach.

Vitamin F deficiency

According to the Danish biochemist, Dr. Jorgen Clausen, multiple sclerosis has a direct connection with the deficiency of unsaturated fatty acids—vitamin F—in the diet. He has demonstrated in animal experiments that when diet is deficient in unsaturated fatty acids, the protective fatty sheaths of *myelin*, which cover the nerves, will be unsufficiently developed; the nerves, not fully protected by this fatty sheath, are more easily subjected to infections of the MS type. In addition to animal experiments, Dr. Clausen has supported his discovery by the geographical occurrence of MS. It has been observed that where diets are deficient in unsaturated fatty acids there is also a higher frequency of multiple sclerosis. Extensive studies made in England show that patients with multiple sclerosis show a much lower blood content of the unsaturated fatty acids than do normal individuals.

Normally, mother's milk, which is richer than cow's milk in unsaturated fatty acids, supplies a sufficient amount of it for the healthy development of the nervous system of a baby. It has been reported that bottle-fed babies have a higher incidence of MS than breast-fed babies. Dr. Clausen has demonstrated that rats fed a diet without unsaturated fats immediately developed symptoms of multiple sclerosis.

DRS. ECKEL AND LUTZ EXPERIMENT

Two Austrian doctors have treated 39 patients over a period of more than two years with a controlled diet. Since MS is essentially a disease of the fatty sheathing of the nerves, they theorized that the disease may be caused by a faulty fat metabolism due to overconsumption of carbohydrates; therefore, the only dietary restriction was practically a total elimination of carbohydrates—no more than 15–20 grams of carbohydrates a day were allowed. This diet did not affect favorably the more advanced cases, but in twelve cases, some of which were recent and some of only a few years' duration, the doctors reported complete or nearly complete recovery.[5] Some corroborative research was done also in the United States on the possible link between a carbohydrate diet (and resultant hypoglycemia) and multiple sclerosis.[6]

EVERS DIET THERAPY

The most successful of all attempts to treat multiple sclerosis are the two dietary methods used extensively in Europe, particularly in Germany—the Evers therapy and the Waerland therapy.

Joseph Evers, M.D., is the founder of the only clinic in the world which specializes in the treatment of multiple sclerosis. He has treated well over 10,000 multiple sclerosis cases in his clinic and has achieved very dramatic results. Patients come from all over the world to Dr. Evers' clinic and in most cases they leave his clinic healed and restored to health. Naturally, advanced cases cannot be helped. If a major portion of the central nervous system is damaged and most of the vital organs affected, nothing can help the patient.

In his excellent books, *The Changed Aspects of Diseases* and *Directions for Treatment of Multiple Sclerosis*,[7] Dr. Evers points out that multiple sclerosis is a metabolic disease caused by faulty nutrition. In the past, man has lived for thousands of years on pure unadulterated natural foods without poisons and toxic chemical substances. Today our foods, because of wrong agricultural methods, processing and chemical additives, contain over 2,000 substances to which man is not adapted and which his system is not able to handle. Dr. Evers specifically points out a replacement of wholesome sourdough whole-meal bread by devitilized white bread, and raw milk by pasteurized and homogenized milk, as some of the most serious assaults on man's natural foods. Thus, denatured foods cause metabolic disorder and are responsible for the many degenerative metabolic diseases, such as obesity, arthritis, diabetes, and a host of other diseases, *including multiple sclerosis.*

Dr. Evers' program

First, all manufactured, canned, processed, refined, frozen, and denatured foods are omitted. Anything made from white flour and white sugar is specifically prohibited, as such foods are lacking in the vital nutrients of vitamins and mineral salts. Coffee, tea, chocolate, salt, sugar, mustard, pepper, and vinegar are also prohibited.

Dr. Evers' patients receive a diet of raw fruits, root vegetables, raw milk, raw eggs, raw rolled oats (freshly prepared and not steamed), honey and water. In addition, the patients receive sprouted seeds* and raw fermented foods, such as sauerkraut,* fermented wheat and fermented dairy products.* In less severe cases, and when the patients are well on their way to recovery (and also in the case of older patients), raw meat is added to their diet. Dr. Evers specifically uses raw ham and raw bacon. He permits an occasional glass of pure wine. As you can see, the emphasis is on *raw* foods.

Dr. Evers also treats with his diets other metabolic diseases, such as leukemia, rheumatoid arthritis, lymphogranulomatosis, and plasmocytoma. He has achieved especially good results in hundreds of cases of infantile muscular dystrophy.

WAERLAND THERAPY

In Chapter 5, I have described Are Waerland's philosophy of natural living. His wife Ebba Waerland is an accomplished practitioner in the application of Waerland therapies in the treatment of many diseases. In her book, *Naturläkekonstens Bok,*[8] she describes dietetic Waerland therapies which she has applied in many clinics in Germany and Sweden in the treatment of multiple sclerosis. They are also described in an English language book by Are Waerland, *Health Is Your Birthright.*[9]

First, Waerland and Evers agree completely as to the cause of multiple sclerosis: a diet of denatured foods which is lacking in important nutritive elements and which causes metabolic disorder and poisons the system. Their general dietetic measures are similiar as well. Ebba Waerland recommends complete removal of all processed, refined, and devitilized foods, as well as sugar, tobacco, alcohol, salt, coffee, tea, spices and other foodless products.

The Waerland therapy for multiple sclerosis

Treatment begins with a short fast of not over five days' duration, with vegetable and fruit juices. After fasting, a strict alkaline diet is prescribed for at least two weeks. This diet consists of two meals a day of raw fruits and vegetables with the addition of sprouted wheat* and 1 slice of whole meal bread; one meal is a vegetable meal, the other a fruit meal. This is followed by the standard Waerland diet (see Chapter 5) with the addition of sprouted wheat. Only unpasteurized, raw milk is permitted. Bread consumption is limited to one or two slices of sour-dough bread a day. Cold-pressed oils are used instead of butter. No cheese, except whey cheese and homemade cottage cheese,* is allowed. Brewer's yeast is recommended as a food supplement.

In addition to the diet, other biological means of detoxifying the system advocated by Ebba Waerland are increasing the blood circulation by massage, exercises, and special hydrotherapeutic treatments.

ADVICE TO MS SUFFERERS

If you suffer from multiple sclerosis, my advice would be to show this chapter—and still better the original books by Evers and Waerland, and other references—to your doctor and ask for his opinion on the advisability of trying the Evers and Waerland therapies in your particular case. Of course, both therapies are completely harmless biological methods and you could not possibly get worse by trying them. They may, in fact, save your life.

You may also benefit by reading *Let's Get Well* by Adelle Davis.[10] She describes several cases of multiple sclerosis helped by applied nutrition and vitamin therapy. She quotes researchers' work in these areas and suggests that heavy doses of vitamins, especially of vitamin E, C, pantothenic acid, B_2 and B_6, plus her so-called Antistress Program, have helped a number of persons to "recover completely from multiple sclerosis." Show her book to your doctor also and ask him if the vitamin therapy advocated by Adelle Davis may be tried in your case.

I hope that this chapter will show hundreds of thousands of sufferers of MS that there is hope for them; that the nutritional approach may have an answer to their problem. Why not try to find an unprejudiced, understanding doctor, preferably nutritionally- and biologically-inclined, who is willing to try an unorthodox approach, and ask him to help you with the application of the knowledge presented in this chapter.

13

How the Latest European Discoveries Can Help You to Grow Hair

From Sweden comes some hopeful and exciting news for the millions of bald and balding men and women around the world.

Lars Engstrand, M.D., assistant professor at the famous Karolinska Medical Institute in Stockholm, has made extensive studies of the problems of pathological conditions in the blood vessel system, particularly of the blood circulation in the small capillaries. By exact measurements of blood distribution to various surfaces of the skin, he observed that blood circulation in the scalp was impaired in men more often than in women. He has worked on the theory developed by the German Doctor Kessler, who found that the enlarged tendinous membrane in men deprived hair follicles of sufficient amounts of fresh blood, thus stopping the production of new hair.

The difference in male and female head crowns (galea)

The crown of the head in both men and women is covered with a thin sheet-like membrane called the *galea*. At the age of 15, this membrane is paper-thin, or about 0.2 millimeters thick, in both sexes. In women, the galeas remains thin and elastic throughout life. But in men, from approximately 16–18 years of age, the galea gradually becomes thicker and loses its elasticity. This continues until the age of 50–55, when it becomes stabilized and remains unchanged for about ten years, after which a degenerative process, linked to old age, sets in and the membrane again becomes thinner (which explains why many bald men suddenly notice some new hair growing on previously bald areas after they reach 65–70).

When the tendinous membrane becomes thick, it increases the pressure and the tension on the scalp and on the blood vessels. This pressure leads to a diminished blood supply to the small blood capillaries, which are located just above this membrane, and which, among other functions, feed the hair follicles with the nutrients necessary for hair growth. The result: a gradual diminishing of hair growth until the hair follicles are unable to produce any more hairs and the skin is left bare.

According to Dr. Engstrand, even an insignificant tension in the thickened membrane will cause a diminished blood supply to the hair follicles. He said that in cases of advanced baldness the membrane can become ten times thicker than its original size and will completely block the distribution of the blood to the small capillaries above the membrane.

Are bald men more sexy?

What causes the galea to become thick? Why do men become bald but not women?

Dr. Engstrand stated that the thickening of the tendinous scalp membrane is effected by the male sex hormones. He indicated several other possible causes for this condition, but the main cause is hormone stimulation. Men with a generous sex hormone production have a greater chance of losing their hair. This explains the typical male pattern of baldness: bald head but otherwise vigorous secondary male sex characteristics—thick, fast-growing beard and abundant hair growth on the other parts of the body.

A hereditary tendency is also indicated. Not only is there a great variety in the quantity of sex hormones produced by different men, but even the amount of blood which each individual, anatomically speaking, has available for his scalp, varies considerably from man to man and is hereditary to some extent. Also, Dr. Engstrand stressed the fact that hormone production and stimulation can vary to a great extent during different periods and various ages of the same individual. In addition, excessive hair loss can be influenced by such factors as nutritional deficiencies and prolonged mental or emotional stress. Mental stress causes tensions in the muscle tissues of the scalp and the neck and thus constricts the blood vessels.

How Dr. Engstrand's theory was proven

Dr. Engstrand developed a special surgical method which he calls The Radical Scalp Operation According to Engstrand. The operation is aimed at relieving the pressure in the scalp by making several incisions in the galea. It is a simple operation without hospitalization which takes about 50 minutes to perform. Dr. Engstrand has performed over 1,000 such operations and reports quite remarkable results. In the most favorable group of patients, between 70 and 80 percent experienced increased hair growth within six months to a year. Even in completely bald areas—in the recessed temples and at the crown of the head—his method has brought new hair growth in 40 to 50 percent of the patients, provided that the baldness was of a shorter duration than five years.

Thus, Dr. Engstrand has definitely proven that loss of hair and baldness is indeed caused by impaired blood circulation. Whether or not the surgical approach is the right and most effective way to increase blood distribution to the hair follicles remains to be seen. In accord with the spirit of this book, which is basically a self-help book, I am inclined to think that there are easier ways than operations to stimulate the increased blood flow to the hair roots. I am referring to the nutritional approach. And in this regard I have very exciting news for you.

CASE HISTORIES

Totally bald man gets full head of hair!

It happened in Stockholm. The man was totally bald for several years—I mean he had no hair whatever on the top of his head. This didn't bother him very much, but he also suffered from hardening of the arteries and atherosclerosis, which was a greater reason for concern. The largest hospital in Sweden, Södersjukhuset in Stockholm, tested new treatments for these diseases. Over one hundred patients participated in prolonged treatments with nicotinic acid, one of the B-vitamins, also called niacin. Our bald man was one of the patients in this test group. After three years of treatment with nicotinic acid he received a vigorous hair growth on his previously bald head and is now the proud owner of a full head of hair.[1]

Nicotinic acid has a widening and dilating effect on blood vessels, particularly on the peripheral capillary system. It would seem that the vigorous hair growth in this case was effected by the increased blood supply through the dilated blood vessels and capillaries in the scalp.

Note: Do not confuse nicotinic acid with nicotine, which is a very dangerous poison and has no relation to nicotinic acid, a B-vitamin.

English doctor cures baldness—unintentionally!

Dr. John Kelvin reported in the British Medical Journal that he treated many patients for blood vessel disorders with the drug composition *beta-pyridylkarbinol,* derivative of vitamin substance *pyridin-3-carbonic acid.* The drug was intended to improve blood circulation in the feet and hands. The doctor noticed that some of his bald patients had new hair growth.

"I didn't connect this new hair growth with the drug I was using until one more of my patients, who had been totally bald previously, walked into my office one morning with a beautiful and well-combed head of hair!" said the doctor.

After this incident was publicized, the English paper reported that the drug stores were stormed by a multitude of men of all ages asking for "the new tablets."

H-PANTOTEN TABLETS FOR HAIR GROWTH

As a consequence of these experiments in Sweden and England, the Swedish Pharmaceutical Company AB Carls-Bergh has put out a vitamin-mineral-trace-element-amino-acid preparation for hair in a tablet form called *H-Pantotén.* The active ingredients in H-Pantotén are: vitamin H (biotin), pantothenic acid, nicotinic acid, folic acid, para-amino-benzoic acid, inositol—all vitamins from B-complex—plus iron, iodine and other trace elements, and some vital amino acids. I have heard several remarkable testimonies by users of this preparation. Here is what Mrs. N. C., 73, from Helsingfors, Finland, writes:

A couple of years ago I bought a bottle of H-Pantotén in a health food store and also some wheat germ. I take two dessert spoons of wheat germ each morning with buttermilk and one Pantotén tablet. This treatment has helped me so much that now I have no use for the wig I was using before. My hair has grown fast and I have long hair now. But you have to keep with it every day . . .

I also had cramps in both legs and even that trouble disappeared. Needless to say, I am very happy. I'd like to add that my hair also got a much better color.

An actor, who tried H-Pantotén writes:

I had my hair tinted and in order to get back the natural color, I shaved my head. But the re-growth was very slow and uneven. Various treatments I tried did not seem to help. A good friend told me about H-Pantotén and I have been using it for over 2 months. My hair is growing fast and vigorously now and it has the original color.

How H-Pantotén works

It has been long recognized that hair is a living part of your body, just as your skin, teeth or nails, and that it must be fed by your blood stream. Your blood can not deliver to your hair all the required nutrients unless it is supplied with all these nutrients from your food. But if your diet is deficient in some of the required vitamins, minerals, trace elements and proteins, then your blood will be deficient in these elements, too, and will not be able to supply them to your hair.

This is self evident—but this is only half of the truth!

It is often said that "you are what you eat," which is also only half of the truth. The fact is that you are not what you eat, but *what you assimilate*. You may eat the most nutritious and best-balanced diet in the world, but if your digestive and assimilative system is out of order and can not assimilate the required nutrients and send them to the blood, then you still can be suffering from malnutrition and nutritional deficiencies.

The same is true in regard to hair growth. Books have been written on the relationship between nutrition and hair growth. You need such and such food factors in order to supply your hair with all the nutritive elements it needs for healthy growth. But if your blood vessels and the small blood capillaries in your scalp are so constricted that they are unable to supply blood to the hair follicles, then even if you eat the best food in the world and take all the extra nutrients required for hair growth in the form of vitamin and mineral supplements, it won't do your hair a bit of good! Unless you improve the blood circulation in the scalp so that the required nutrients will be able to get to the hair roots, all your attempts to "feed your hair from within" will be futile.

That's why the Swedish H-Pantotén tablets have been so successful. Not only do they contain the vital nutritive elements, known to science today to be essential for healthy hair growth, but they also contain certain B-complex vitamins known to be able to dilate the blood vessels so that these nutrients can travel through the blood stream to the hair roots.

FACTS AND FALLACIES
ABOUT NUTRITION FOR HAIR GROWTH

I will discuss all the nutritive factors connected with better hair growth, or, in reverse, the nutritional deficiencies connected with hair loss and baldness, later in this chapter. But first let me disprove one of the fallacious notions held by many authorities on the hair-through-nutrition subject. They claim that for healthy hair growth you need first and foremost *"protein, protein and more protein."*

In Chapter 6 I have tried to discredit the high protein myth. Of course it is true that just about all your body is made up of protein. Of course it is true that your *hair* is also made up largely of protein. But this does not mean that you have to eat masses of protein each day. Your actual protein need for the normal, healthy functioning of all the vital organs and processes of your body is only about 30 grams a day, which can be supplied by one pint of milk and a cheese sandwich. Protein intake should not exceed 50–60 grams per day—which is less than half what is usually advocated in the United States. Proteins eaten in excess of the actual need, especially animal proteins, are definitely detrimental to your health, including the health of your hair. And don't forget that practically *all* natural foods contain some protein, even fruits and vegetables.

Here is something to ponder: Are there many bald heads in Japan, China, India, or Mexico? In these countries a bald man is rare and the hair retains its blue-black color until very old age. Yet these people live, by American standards, on a very low protein diet. Certainly, hereditary factors have some part to play in this. But heredity is not the whole answer, as demonstrated by the fact that Chinese and Mexicans get gray hair and even become sleek-bald when they move to the United States and adopt western habits of eating. Studies of the nutritional habits of these people have shown that their diets are very high in vitamins, especially vitamins C and B; minerals; trace elements, especially iodine; and essential fatty acids—all very important for healthy hair growth.

If you'd like to undertake a program of feeding your hair from within, please don't stuff yourself with huge amounts of animal protein. Too much animal protein may cause metabolic disorders, self-intoxication and hardening of the arteries with resultant impaired blood circulation—in other words, it may create the very problems you are trying to remedy. *Enough, but not too much, should be the rule in regard to protein.*

OPTIMUM NUTRITION FOR HAIR GROWTH

If you have problems of hair loss you should first see that your general health is well taken care of. Various derangements in the functions of your vital organs must be corrected. The digestive system must be in good working condition, so that the nutrients from the foods you eat will be properly assimilated. Also, see that the glandular system, particularly the thyroid gland, is active and that the nervous system is working well. It is worthwhile to have a thorough physical check-up to be sure that there are no pathological conditions as an underlying cause for the hair loss.

From the point of view of hair loss and baldness, there are certain nutritive elements which have been found to have a direct relation to the health of the hair. These are as follows:

B-complex vitamins

Vitamin B is one of the most important vitamins for your hair.

It has been demonstrated that the two of the most important B-vitamins for hair growth are *inositol* and *choline*. The other B-vitamins, pantothenic acid, para-amino-benzolic acid and folic acid, have been also linked with hair loss, and particularly with the graying of the hair. Animal tests have shown that these vitamins can restore the natural color to the hair. This has been also reported by many men using these vitamins.

Biotin, also known as vitamin H, is necessary for the normal metabolism of proteins and fats in the system. Biotin deficiency has been shown to cause fat dandruff which contributes to the loss of hair. It has been demonstrated in animal experiments that if biotin is totally removed from the diet, the animals lose their hair. When biotin is added again to their diet, the condition of their fur is soon improved.

In human beings, biotin deficiency has resulted in seborrhea, lack of appetite, skin disorders and inflammations. It is believed that the daily requirement of this vitamin is 150 to 300 micrograms.

Pantothenic acid deficiency in men has caused, among other things, chronic fatigue, increased tendency for infections and loss of hair. The daily requirement is 8–10 mg.

Niacin, or *nicotinic acid,* has a blood vessel dilating property; it is especially effective in widening the small peripheral blood capillaries. This is of vital importance for getting nutrition to the hair roots. The daily requirement is approximately 15 mg.

Vitamin B_9, or *folic acid,* is extremely important for the health of the skin. Folic acid deficiency can cause serious skin disorders. Persons deficient in folic acid often become completely bald. When folic acid is introduced back into the diet, hair starts to grow normally.

Inositol is vital also for hair growth. It works together with pantothenic acid and choline and is involved in vital metabolic processes. A diet low in inositol can cause hair to fall out. Some authorities advise taking 3,000 mg. or half a teaspoon of inositol daily.

Deficiencies of vitamins B_2 (*riboflavin*) and B_6 (*pyridoxine*) have also been shown to cause impaired hair growth.

As you can see, almost all vitamins from B-complex are involved in one way or another in the loss of hair and baldness.

How to take B-vitamins for hair growth

For your hair's sake, do not rush to your nearest drug store and buy the pure, isolated B-vitamins mentioned above. There is danger involved in taking large doses of synthetic B-vitamins separately. Taking one B-vitamin separately may cause a deficiency of another B vitamin. For example, taking large amounts of niacin may cause a deficiency of thiamin (B_1). In fact it is known through animal tests that taking single synthetic B-vitamins may result in the directly opposite effect than that hoped for—impaired health generally and weakened hair growth. Furthermore, the two of the B-vitamins which are vitally important for the health of your hair, folic acid and para-amino-benzoic acid, are now sold only on prescription in the United States.

The best way to assure that you get all the B-vitamins named above without the risk of overdosage or imbalance, is to take only a natural B-vitamin preparation, sold usually through health food stores. Practically all manufacturers of natural vitamins have a B-complex formula. Read the labels and select the formula with all the B-vitamins discussed in this chapter. See that the formula contains particularly large amounts of biotin, choline and inositol; also pantothenic acid, nicotinic acid, and folic acid. Take B-complex tablets as directed on the bottle. In addition, the following five food supplements contain B-complex vitamins in well-blended and biologically potent combination:

- Brewer's yeast (powder and tablets) —up to two tablespoons a day, or the equivalent in tablets.
- Desiccated liver (powder or tablets) —five to ten tablets a day.
- Lecithin (granules or liquid) —one to two tablespoons a day.
- Wheat germ (raw) —two to three tablespoons a day.
- Sunflower seeds (whole or meal) —two tablespoons a day.

These food supplements are the richest known natural sources of the B-complex vitamins. In addition, they are rich in other vital nutritional elements, such as enzymes, minerals, trace elements, and—last but not least—they are an excellent source of the complete proteins. Desiccated liver is also rich in iron and copper, the deficiency of which has been shown to cause anemia with resultant hair loss, as demonstrated by Swedish researcher Dr. S. Hard.[2]

That iron deficiency can cause hair loss has been also observed in St. George Hospital in London. Two women blood donors started to lose their hair. When they were given iron supplements, their hair condition returned to normal.

Vitamins and food supplements should be taken with foods, divided equally among three meals.

Vitamin E

Vitamin E has been shown to have hair-growth-promoting properties.

In experiments with rats, conducted by two Japanese researchers, it has been demonstrated that topical application of vitamin E made hair grow 2.4 times faster than normal.[3] Vitamin E works by increasing the blood flow to the skin surface, causing a rise in skin temperature and an increase in blood volume. Vitamin E is also effective

taken internally. It oxygenates the blood and stimulates the circulation.

Wheat germ (rich in vitamins B and E) and wheat germ oil
(the richest natural source of vitamin E) are used extensively in the
fur-animal industry. Mink and fox growers have used these foods for
years because they give a healthy, thick and luxuriant fur to their
animals.

One tablespoon of wheat germ oil, two to three tablespoons of
raw wheat germ, and/or 300 to 600 I.U. of vitamin E in capsule
form, are the usually recommended doses.

Vitamin C and bioflavonoids

Vitamin C is such an universal wonder vitamin that it should be
routinely prescribed in every condition of ill health. Vitamin C plays
an important role in the health of all connective tissues. It is linked
to the health and proper functioning of the adrenal glands. Bioflavonoids (or vitamin P) which always accompany vitamin C in its
natural form are known to be essential for the healthy condition of
the blood capillaries.

Health food stores usually stock organic forms of vitamin C
with bioflavonoids from which you make your selection.

Vitamin F

Vitamin F, found in essential fatty acids, is considered by many
European doctors to be a very important factor for a healthy scalp
and good hair growth. The condition of the sebaceous glands, which
are located in and around the hair follicles, is closely related to the
health of the hair. The sebaceous glands produce an oily secretion,
sebum, which lubricates the scalp and hair and moisturizes the skin.
Vitamin F is considered essential for the healthy condition of the
sebaceous glands.

The best sources of essential fatty acids are cold-pressed, unrefined vegetable oils, which may be purchased at most health food
stores.

Vitamin A

Also vitamin A is universally acknowledged for its great beneficial effect on the health of the skin. Since many hair conditions are
connected with excessive dandruff and dry, itchy, and flaky scalp,
vitamin A can be of considerable benefit in such conditions.

The richest source of natural vitamin A is cod liver oil. One or two teaspoons of cod liver oil will supply you with good amounts of vitamins A, D and E, and with unsaturated fatty acids.

OTHER FACTORS TO PROMOTE HAIR GROWTH

All *minerals* are important for the health of the hair, especially calcium, magnesium, potassium, phosphorus, iron, copper, and iodine. Vitamin D (cod liver oil) is important for the proper assimilation of the minerals in the intestines. (*Remember:* you are not what you *eat*, but what you *assimilate*.)

Iodine is a trace mineral which is found in foods and water in extremely small quantities. It is needed by the thyroid for its healthy functioning. It has been observed that iodine deficiency in the diet causes dryness, thinness and poor growth of hair. Iodine has a direct action on the activity of the thyroid gland. When the thyroid gland is functioning to its fullest capacity, the general metabolism is speeded up, which has a favorable effect on the quality and growth of the hair. It is also believed that iodine has something to do with keeping hair from turning gray.

The best natural source of iodine is kelp. Kelp is a dried and powdered seaweed, and can be obtained from health food stores in tablet or powder form. One or two kelp tablets usually contain a minimum daily requirement of iodine.

Remember that the diets of people known for their healthy, thick hair—the Chinese, Italians, Japanese, Eskimos, etc.—are rich in iodine, which is procured from sea foods and seaweed. Seaweed is a staple food in many countries, notably in Japan.

A few years ago sheep farmers in the Great Lakes region complained that they were having trouble growing wool on their sheep. Iodine is lacking in the soils of this area, as in many other inland regions of the United States. When the farmers added iodine to the sheep's rations, the quality and quantity of wool improved immediately.

Kelp is also rich in many other minerals necessary for healthy hair growth, such as calcium, magnesium, phosphorus, and potassium. One or two kelp tablets with each meal is a good protective dosage.

Lecithin is very rich in choline, inositol, and phosphorus—all acknowledged hair-growth stimulants. Lecithin is a modern wonder food, indeed, and much scientific research is available which shows that it is essential for many vital functions of the body. It is extremely important for the health of the nerves. It is vital for the brain—28 percent of the brain is lecithin. It is credited with the ability to break up fat and prevent fatty deposits in the arteries—one of the plagues of modern man. It rejuvenates the endocrinal glands which are involved in the growth of hair.

Commercial lecithin, available at health food stores, is made from soybeans. It comes in granular, liquid, or tablet form. Take two to three teaspoons, or the equivalent in tablets, each day.

DON'TS OF THE HAIR-FROM-WITHIN PROGRAM

In addition to the positive factors named above for the prevention of baldness and for the stimulation of hair growth, here are some negative ones. Avoid the following: salt; white sugar and white flour; excessive amounts of animal fats; alcohol and smoking; prolonged emotional stress.

Experiments conducted in Sweden indicate that cutting down *salt* in the diet will significantly reduce hair loss. The American scientist, Dr. Eugene Foldes, of New York, has in his experiments arrived at similar conclusions.[4]

White sugar and *white flour* and all foods or beverages made with them are not only worthless from a nutritional point of view, but they are definitely health destroyers. From the originally good natural products, sugar beets, sugar cane and whole wheat, virtually all the nutritive elements have been removed. What remains is nothing but pure starch, which you certainly don't need to grow hair. What is even worse, sugar and white flour destroy B-vitamins in your system—the very vitamins that you have learned a few pages back are so vital for the healthy condition of your hair.

Alcohol is pure carbohydrate and also destroys B vitamins in your body.

Tobacco constricts blood capillaries and robs your system of vitamin C: both important factors connected with hair loss. It has been proven by extensive research performed by Dr. J. H. Burn, of Oxford, that smoking constricts the arteries and small capillaries, and slows down blood circulation.

Excessive amounts of *animal fats* and refined carbohydrates in the diet can adversely affect the normal functioning of the sebaceous glands, as has been found by the famed dermatologist Dr. Lubowe. Replace animal fats and hydrogenated fats in your diet with cold-pressed unsaturated vegetable oils, such as corn oil, safflower oil, wheat germ oil, olive oil, etc., all also rich in essential fatty acids and vitamin E.

Avoid *prolonged emotional* and *mental stress.* Emotional stress causes constriction of the blood vessels of the scalp and tensions in the muscle tissues. This will block the narrow blood capillaries of the scalp and prevent blood from coming to the roots of the hair.

TEN-POINT DO-IT-YOURSELF PROGRAM
FOR BETTER HAIR GROWTH

To sum up the information in this chapter, here is a do-it-yourself program to stimulate your hair growth and prevent hair loss and baldness—and possibly even grow new hair on already bald heads!

1. *H-Pantotén* tablets are made in Sweden and are sold in every drug store, health food store and barber shop in Sweden and also in many other countries on the European continent. Perhaps they will soon be available in the United States. If you can obtain them, take one to three tablets each day, preferably before breakfast. If you are not able to obtain *H-Pantotén,* use a natural, multiple high-potency B-complex vitamin formula. Health food stores have several to choose from. Select one which has all the B-vitamins present with especially large doses of those B-vitamins named in this chapter as being of particular importance for the hair and for improving blood circulation: inositol, choline, biotin, pantothenic acid, nicotinic acid, folic acid, riboflavin, and pyridoxine. Take B-complex formulas before breakfast and before dinner.

2. Supplement your diet with a varied choice of the following B-vitamin-packed foods:
   - Brewer's yeast—one to two tablespoons a day.
   - Desiccated liver (important for B_{12})—five to ten tablets a day.
   - Lecithin—one to two tablespoons a day.
   - Wheat germ—two to three tablespoons a day.
   - Sunflower seeds, whole grains, raw nuts, beans. Sunflower seeds are extremely rich in the minerals and vitamins es-

sential for hair growth: choline, inositol, vitamin E and D, and minerals phosphorus, magnesium, and potassium.

3. Take the following additional food supplements:
   - Wheat germ oil—two to three teaspoons a day.
   - Vitamin E—300–600 International Units a day. Start with 100 I.U. and add 100 I.U. each week. (In case of high blood pressure, consult your doctor.)
   - Vitamin C—up to 1,000 mg. a day.
   - Bioflavonoids—20–100 mg. a day.
   - Cold-pressed vegetable oils—use them liberally with your salads or in cooking.
   - Cod liver oil—one tsp. daily.
   - Kelp—one tablet with each meal.
   - Bone meal tablets, for minerals—five to ten daily.

   Where not suggested otherwise, food supplements should be taken with meals.

4. Eat a balanced diet of vital, natural, unrefined foods, with emphasis on raw fruits and vegetables, nuts, grains, seeds, and milk products.

5. Don't overeat. Hardening of the arteries, which often accompanies obesity, may be a contributing cause of impaired blood circulation and diminished blood supply to your scalp.

6. Avoid salt, white sugar, white flour, and all foods made with them. Use sea salt moderately.

7. Avoid alcohol and tobacco.

8. Avoid excessive shampooing of your hair. Unless your hair is excessively oily, do not wash it oftener than once a week. Vigorous brushing twice a day for a few minutes will normally keep your scalp clean from dirt, dandruff, stale oils, etc. The normal discharge of sebum, the oil from the sebaceous glands, is beneficial for your hair. Vigorous brushing is extremely important for the healthy state of your hair and for the prevention of baldness. It stimulates the sebaceous glands and hair roots and increases the blood supply to the hair follicles.

9. Use finger or vibrator massage to improve blood circulation in your scalp. Here's how you do it: place both hands, all finger tips, firmly on your head and, without moving the fingers, push the whole scalp in circular movements for a few seconds; then place the fingers in a new position and

repeat. Cover the whole scalp, including the forehead, temples, and neck. For effortless massage use an electric vibrator, available at department stores for less than ten dollars.

10. Use a slant board or headstand stool, both available at better health food stores. Lie on the slant board, with your head down at the lower level, at least twice a day for 15 minutes each time. If possible, do a headstand twice a day, one to three minutes each time. Both are extremely effective in bringing more blood to the blood-starving scalp. Many men have reported better hair growth and even new hair in completely bald areas after practicing headstands for a few months.

Warning: If you suffer from high blood pressure, or if your blood capillaries are in poor shape and brittle, build up your condition and strengthen your capillaries with the vitamins C, P and the macrobiotic diet outlined in Chapter 15 before attempting headstands.

14

How to Keep Young
with Miracle Foods from the Bees

*From their bellies (the bees)
comes a liquor which is medicine for man.*
—*The Koran*

There are 21,708 people in the Soviet Union who are over 100 years old, according to the 1959 census. And there are quite a few who have reached the respectable age of 150 and over.

Some years ago the famed Russian scientist, biologist and experimental botanist, Dr. Nicolai Tsitsin, was engaged in research on longevity. The aim of his inquiry was to find out ways of prolonging human life.

"We decided to send letters to 200 people claiming to be over 100 years old with the request to answer the following three questions: what was their age, how had they earned their living most of their lives, and what had been their principle food."

Dr. Tsitsin received 150 replies to his 200 letters.

"We made a very interesting discovery. The answers showed that a large number of them were bee-keepers. And *all of them*, without exception, said that their principal food always had been honey!"

But as sensational as this discovery was, this was not all!

"We found," continued Dr. Tsitsin, "that in each case it wasn't really honey these people ate, but the waste matter in the bottom of the beehive. They were poor and they sold all the pure honey on the market, and kept only the dirty residue for themselves."

After a series of laboratory experiments and tests, Dr. Tsitsin discovered that the "dirty residue" of the honey scrap was neither dirt nor honey, but almost pure pollen, which falls off the bees' legs while they deposit their honey. Tsitsin was on the verge of a great nutritional discovery!

HONEY AND POLLEN—HEAVENLY FOODS!

Since time immemorial man has regarded honey and pollen as ambrosia—the food of the gods. Honey is mentioned in the Bible as a specially blessed food. In cave paintings from the Neolithic age (about 15,000 years ago) are illustrations of honey combs being gathered for food. Honey has been found in 3,000-year-old Egyptian pyramids. Pythagoras, a great Greek scientist (600 B.C.), recommended honey for health and long life. Throughout the ages honey has been regarded as a divine food with age-retarding and rejuvenating properties.

The miraculous powers of pollen were also recognized by man in the early ages. Ancient texts from Egypt, Persia and China refer to it. Greek philosophers claimed that pollen held the secret of eternal youth. Pollen was revered as nature's own propagator of life. Raw, unstrained honey, with large proportions of pollen, was used by the original Olympic athletes for extra energy and vitality.

WHAT IS POLLEN?

Pollen is the male germ cells of the plant kingdom. Pollen in beehives and honey comes from flowers. It is believed that it comes to the beehive in two ways: it attaches itself to the legs of honey-collecting bees and then falls off their legs while they deposit their honey; also it is believed that it is deliberately collected by the bees to feed the young working bees which produce royal jelly—another amazing substance on which the queen bee lives exclusively.

Analysis of pollen has shown that it is indeed a food for gods—it is the richest and most complete food in nature!

Pollen contains 20 percent protein; all the water-soluble vitamins (with the exception of B_{12}); a rich supply of minerals and trace elements, and enzymes and coenzymes. The other vital substances are so-called *deoxiribosides* and *sterines,* plus traces of steroid hormone substances and other plant hormones. Most researchers believe, however, that there must be some other as yet undiscovered substances in pollen which must share the credit for its acknowledged prophylactic and therapeutic value. It has been demonstrated that pollen does increase the body's own immunity and also stimulates and rejuvenates glandular activity.

Pollen for prostate trouble

Extensive studies were made by three Swedish doctors, Professor Gösta Jonsson, Dr. Gösta Leander and Professor H. Palmstierna. They reported that strictly controlled tests on 179 cases of chronic prostate inflammation showed that *Cernilton,* a pollen preparation, together with conventional treatments gives in 60 to 80 percent of the cases better results than conventional therapy alone. By 1965 their studies included over 1,100 cases, with the same positive results.

Pollen for hemmorrhoids

Dr. Lars-Erik Essén from Sweden reports that he has used a pollen preparation, Cernitory, for the treatment of hemmorroids. He said that in many cases where treatments with the traditional chemical suppositories were ineffective, the pollen preparation brought about fast relief, even in advanced cases. The preparation is available without prescription in Swedish drug stores.

Pollen for a healthier digestive tract

Many researchers suggest that pollen has an extremely beneficial effect on the digestive tract and intestines. A French researcher, Dr. Remy Chauvin, reports that pollen seems to have an anti-putrefactive factor. It destroys harmful bacteria in the intestines and improves assimilation and elimination. In clinical tests the administration of pollen has relieved chronic constipation and colonic infection. Patients suffering from chronic diarrhea have also showed improvement.

·   It has been suggested that Bulgarians, Rumanians, Russians, and other East European peoples known for their enviable record of longevity have to thank *lactic acid* for their excellent health and youthful vitality. Their diets are high in soured foods (rich in lactic acid), such as sour milk, yogurt, black sour-dough bread, sauerkraut, and the like. Lactic acid has a beneficial anti-putrefactive effect on intestines and keeps the digestive tract in good health.

Probably the most beneficial effect of pollen is that, taken internally, it quickly produces the same anti-putrefactive effect as lactic-acid foods, and thus contributes to a healthy digestive system and good assimilation of nutrients—absolute prerequisites for good health and long life.

Other indications

Pollen in pure form or in the form of Swedish Cernitin preparations has also been used successfully for the following conditions:
- As a general tonic, especially in convalescence and in conditions of neurasthenia.[1]
- In chronic bronchitis, asthma, multiple sclerosis, gastric ulcers, and arthritis.[2]
- In hay fever.[3]
- In treatment of symptoms of aging.[4]

Pollen completely harmless

French doctor Remy Chauvin fed hundreds of experimental mice nothing but pollen for two years to discover possible harmful effects from pollen. Not only he did not see any adverse effects, but through several generations of mice there were increasing vitality and greater reproduction. He continued similiar experiments with children, adults, and old people. There has never been reported any example of the possible harmful effect of pollen on human beings.

TWO REMARKABLE CASES OF RECOVERY

Mrs. Jytte Elmgaard, 35, from Denmark, was stricken by *leuco-encephatalis*—an organic nerve disease with epileptic attacks—in 1950. The disease is considered incurable. During the next ten years her condition grew progressively worse, until by 1961 she was totally paralyzed and bedridden. She had up to 40 epileptic attacks a day, became blind and could not move any part of her body. She lost weight and was fading away fast. No one expected her to survive . . . except her husband who didn't want to give up.

A Danish doctor suggested trying pollen. He obtained a German pollen preparation in liquid form. Mrs. Elmgaard felt some improvement, but not much. A Swedish specialist was consulted and he advised trying *Cernitin T.60* in the form of injections. Injection treatments started in May, 1963, first given by the doctor, then continued by Mr. Elmgaard. The Danish Medical Society gave permission to use these injections and the treatment was at all times under her doctor's supervision. Later, several other pollen preparations were included in the treatment, such as Cernimult, Cernilton, Pollitabs, Polloton 25.

Swedish health magazine Tidskrift för Hälsa, reported three years later that Mrs. Elmgaard has miraculously returned to life. Her condition has been steadily improving. Her vision has returned, she can sit up in her bed and talk, and her paralysis has been disappearing gradually from various parts of her body. Even her weight has become normal. She has to continue with the pollen injections, which in her case seem to have the similar effect that insulin has on a diabetic. The injections keep her free from attacks and improve her general condition.

Doctors were amazed by the "miracle." They could not believe that she was still alive. Her case was reported and widely discussed in medical literature. Doctors suggested, of course, that "certain cases of leucoencephatalis for some unknown reason can heal spontaneously."

Another case is the dramatic case of U.S. Air Force Lt. Col. Thomas J. Tretheway.[5] During World War II, Col. Tretheway spent nine months in a Japanese prison camp as a prisoner of war. His health was in a deplorable state and his weight dropped from 175 pounds to only 85 pounds.

One night he managed to escape. But he was lost in the jungle and finally, after about three days of wandering and with gangrene on his feet, he succumbed to weakness and malnutrition. He was found unconscious by natives of a Chinese jungle tribe.

The natives brought him to the village and treated him for several weeks with a diet rich in pollen and honey. They also coated his feet with pollen and honey. After a few weeks his strength was restored and he was able to walk. The natives guided him to the English lines. An English doctor in Calcutta told him that it was pollen and honey he was to thank for his life and the use of his feet.

Col. Tretheway reported that the natives who saved his life collected pollen from the surface of the water where it had been carried by the wind. They made cakes from it, mixing it with honey—this was their staple diet. They were tall and lean, had perfect teeth, and both children and adults seemed to be in excellent health.

THE ROYAL JELLY

There is another miracle food from the bees that has stirred the imagination of nutritionists and doctors alike—the *royal jelly*.

Royal jelly is the food produced by the worker bees to feed the queen bee. As you probably know, bees have a highly organized community life, with their own systems of mathematics, geography and communications. This community is so well organized and so effectively governed that it is able to collect incredible amounts of food—pollen and honey—during one short summer season. The queen bee is the mother and the sole ruler of the entire hive.

All bees are hatched from eggs, including the queen bee. For the first two or three days after hatching all eggs are fed royal jelly. Then one egg is selected to become queen and she continues to receive royal jelly throughout the rest of her life. The other bees feed themselves on honey.

Now, listen to this: although hatched from similar eggs, the bees fed on honey mature in 21 to 24 days, but the queen bee fed royal jelly is fullgrown in 16 days. The worker bees live an average of two to six months, while the queen bee may live as long as eight years! During this time she works hard at producing eggs. The queen bee lays as many as a quarter of a million eggs in a season, often more than 2,000 eggs in a single day—which is greater than her own weight! Since the queen bee and the worker bees are hatched from identical eggs, it is obvious that the only reason for the great difference in longevity and the marvelous fertility is the difference in the food they eat. Royal jelly must contain a powerful substance or substances able to give the queen bee this enormous energy, fertility and longevity!

Scientists have been trying to find and identify these substances for hundreds of years. So far their efforts have been unsuccessful. Royal jelly does contain all the usual vital factors, which can be isolated: proteins, vitamins, enzymes, etc. It has, however, less of some vitamins than pollen has; and some vitamins, like A for example, are totally missing. Also, little or no vitamin E was found in royal jelly, and the same was true of vitamin C.

However, royal jelly contains more pantothenic acid, one of the B vitamins, than any other known natural substance—up to six times more than brewer's yeast and liver.[6] In experiments reported in the *Journal of Gerontology,* fruit flies were fed royal jelly and their life span was markedly increased. Researchers felt that it was because of the pantothenic acid in royal jelly.

Everyone agrees that royal jelly has marvelous healing and rejuvenating powers, but no one knows why. Feeding control animals *all* the known factors of royal jelly did not bring at all the effects of royal jelly. So, royal jelly obviously contains some other factors which science has not yet been able to detect. Researchers report that all attempts to analyze royal jelly have failed. About 97 to 98 percent of the total has been analyzed and isolated, but the real source of power may be in the remaining elusive two or three percent.

Prophylactic and therapeutic value of royal jelly

An extensive research on royal jelly was made in Czechoslovakia by Dr. Josef Vittek, biologist, and Dr. Jaroslav Kresanek, pharmacologist, at the Medical School in Bratislava. They conducted a five-year investigation and their results are quite remarkable.

- They fed royal jelly in various amounts to test animals and found that it *speeded up their growth and increased their resistance to disease.*[7]
- Royal jelly had an *anti-bacterial* and *anti-virus action,* particularly against *streptococcus,* B. *Coli* and *staphylococcus.*
- Hens, fed royal jelly, increased their egg-laying capacity 20 to 100 percent!
- Royal jelly accelerated the formation of bone tissue.
- Topical application of royal jelly helped to heal wounds in half the time.[8]

Other researchers have reported on royal jelly's preventive effect on cancer. A group of mice were inoculated with four different types of cancerous cells. Half of them were given royal jelly; the other half was used as the control group. While all the mice in the control group died of cancer, the animals fed royal jelly did not show any disorder at all![9]

In the experiments on human beings, Drs. Vittek and Kresanek showed that royal jelly has a favorable influence on body functioning and healing processes in many conditions. Serum cholesterol levels were lowered by the administration of royal jelly for ten days. Royal jelly has shown good results in the treatment of diseases of aging, such as hardening of the arteries, vascular disorders and Buerger's

Disease. German doctors reported that royal jelly preparations showed "satisfactory results" in post-operative conditions. Researchers agreed that royal jelly has a stimulative action upon the functioning of various organs and improves "their associative and coordinative faculties."

However, in spite of some enthusiastic researchers, mostly in Europe, medical science at large has remained skeptical of royal jelly, and virtually no research is being done now to determine its prophylactic and therapeutic possibilities. In the meantime, there are thousands of people, both here and in Europe, who use royal jelly regularly and are satisfied that they benefit from it.

HONEY—MEDICINE OR FOOD?

The answer to the above question is both! More than any other food, honey fulfills Hippocrates' requirement for an ideal food: i.e., that "our food must be our medicine—our medicine must be our food."

As a food, honey is vastly superior to white sugar. Honey was man's natural sweetener for thousands of years, until he discovered how to make a cheaper artificial sweetener—sugar. For this discovery man has paid with more suffering in terms of ill health than for any other of his attempts to improve on nature, with the possible exception of his discovery of cooking!

White sugar is completely void of any nutritional value, with the exception of chemically pure carbohydrate.

Honey, on the other hand, is a perfect food. In addition to the easy assimilable form of sugar, it contains large amounts of vitamins and minerals, being particularly rich in vitamins B and C. It contains practically all of the vitamins of the B-complex, which are needed in the system for the digestion and metabolism of sugar. Honey is also rich in minerals, such as calcium, phosphorus, sodium, magnesium, potassium, silicon, etc. This is specifically true of the darker varieties of honey, such as buckwheat honey.

The vitamin C content of honey varies considerably, depending on the source of the nectar. Some kinds may contain as much as 300 milligrams of vitamin C per 100 grams of honey.

The natural sugars in honey are easily digested, as they are in a pre-digested form, converted to that state by the enzymatic action of the bees' salivary glands.

Honey is an alkaline food. It contains organic acids, similar to the acids of fruits, which produce alkalinity in the system through the body's chemistry. Since the average diet tends to be too acid-forming, it is of importance that you eat as many alkaline foods as possible.

Honey as medicine

As a medicine, honey was and still is credited with marvelous curative powers. A whole book could be written on all the medicinal uses of honey, from the thousands of years of folk medicine to the scientific research of the present time. It is sufficient here to say that in addition to definite age-retarding properties honey has been proven to be from mildly beneficial to extraordinarily effective in the following conditions:

- It increases calcium retention (as compared with sugar) in infant feeding.[10]
- It increases hemoglobin count and can prevent or cure nutritional anemia; honey is rich in iron and copper.
- It is an excellent mild laxative, especially recommended as such for infants and children.
- It has been shown to be useful in rheumatic and arthritic conditions, especially in combination with apple cider vinegar (Dr. D. C. Jarvis, M.D.) .
- It has been used successfully in the treatment of liver and kidney disorders, diseases of the respiratory and digestive tracts, weak heart action, infectious diseases, colds, insomnia, poor circulation, and bad complexion.
- Applied externally on ulcers and sores it speeds the healing processes. It is one of nature's best bacteria-destroying agents.
- German researchers have found that hay fever is relieved by eating honey which contains pollen to which patients are allergic! Also asthma, related to hay fever, is improved by eating honey.

HOW TO STAY YOUNGER LONGER WITH THE MIRACLE FOODS FROM THE BEES

You have seen in this chapter that foods from the bees—honey, pollen and royal jelly—do indeed have great potentials for health and longevity. It would be unwise to ignore these foods which have been used with so great a benefit by the ancients. In the terms of practical application of the information in this chapter you can do the following:

1. Pollen and pollen preparations are available in the United States in the better health food stores. So are the preparations containing royal jelly. It certainly would not hurt to try these—and you just may be surprised by the benefits. Specifically in conditions of intestinal sluggishness and putrefaction in the digestive tract, pollen has definitely proven to be exceedingly beneficial.

2. Honey, pollen, and royal jelly are definitely rejuvenating, age-retarding foods. They have a stimulating effect on all the vital processes of your body. Follow the example of Russian centenarians and use them liberally—and see yourself growing younger as the symptoms of old age gradually disappear.

3. Stop using white sugar! Replace it with health-giving honey. Honey can be used everywhere sugar is used: in beverages, in baking, in cooking, on cereals, etc. We have a double reason to use honey instead of sugar—honey is so inexpensive here! In most European countries honey costs two to three times more than it does here. And, in spite of the food industry's efforts to "improve" on nature, honey is still one of the least-tampered-with natural foods you can buy.

4. Use only raw, unheated and unstrained honey. Heating destroys both vitamins and enzymes. Refining, filtering and "clarifying" of honey removes many of the minerals and amino acids—yes, honey even contains amino acids, the essential forms of protein! And what is even worse, refining and filtering removes the pollen! Also, choose the dark varieties of honey in preference to the light; dark honey contains more vitamin and minerals than light-colored honey.

Remember: The miracle foods from the bees—honey, pollen and royal jelly—will give you many health benefits and will keep you younger longer. After all, they have been used for these purposes for many thousands of years!

15

The Secrets of Staying Healthfully Young — European Style

If you have good health you are young.
—English Proverb

The diseases of old age are not due to old age; they are due to wrong life.
—J. H. Tilden, M.D.

Men have sought the fountain of youth since the dawn of history. The medicine man of the Stone Age, in addition to being a specialist in driving the evil spirits away, also tried to restore virility to aging men. Records from early medical history show a variety of herbs used to retard aging processes and revitalize aging bodies. In the Orient, magic rejuvenating properties were attributed to ginseng, the root with a resemblance to the human figure. The Papyrus of Eber, the oldest medical document known, describes the use of animal organs for virility and long life. The Hindu doctor Susrata, 1400 B.C., prescribed tiger's sex glands for men suffering from loss of potency. Chinese doctors of the third century used placental tissue as a rejuvenating tonic.

Interest in methods of preventing premature aging and staying younger longer has never been as keen as it is at the present time. The second half of the twentieth century will be known in history as the era of the worship of youth. Modern men and women go to great lengths in their efforts to prevent premature aging and not only to feel but also to look younger. Also, modern science is engaged in a search for ways of prolonging man's life and preventing the diseases and symptoms of aging. A special branch of medical science, *gerontology*, is busy working to solve the secrets of aging and find ways of prolonging life. Many startling discoveries have already been made in various parts of the world. Let me share with you some of the newest European facts and discoveries in the art of staying young.

REJUVENATION SWEDISH STYLE

Swedish women, internationally known for their luscious complexions and youthful beauty, use certain natural foods to stay beautiful.

Swedish beauty secret number one—rose hips—is also Swedish rejuvenation secret number one: *Rose hips tea is the Swedish fountain of youth!*

Here's how rose hips can keep you young. Russian scientists have discovered that vitamin C has a profound stimulating effect on the adrenal glands. Adrenal glands secrete over 20 steroid hormones which are directly involved in keeping your vital bodily processes in a condition of high efficiency. It is generally agreed that a decrease in the output of these hormones, which usually begins in late middle life, is responsible for the symptoms of aging. Russian researchers have demonstrated that substantial daily doses of vitamin C have a rejuvenating, stimulating effect on the glandular activity, and the vital hormones are once more produced at higher levels, similar to the level of younger people.

Vitamin C is also known to play an essential part in the oxidation-reduction system of tissue respiration, as shown by Dr. W. J. McCormick, M.D. In addition, vitamin C is a known chemotherapeutic agent; in fact it is the most potent natural "drug" known in the therapy of practically all bacterial and viral infections. Vitamin C is also a highly potent anti-toxic agent and protects the body from all kinds of poisonous substances, both those originating within the system, as a result of sluggish digestion and elimination, as well as those introduced into the system by food, water and air. Since growing old is often associated with sluggish metabolism and autointoxication, it is easy to see how large doses of vitamin C can have a rejuvenating effect on old people.

There is also growing evidence that the aging process is largely a matter of the diminished oxygenation of the cells. Vitamin C has a great effect on improved cell breathing and thus prevents premature aging.

Perhaps the most vital function of vitamin C is in keeping collagen, the cellular cement, healthy. The visible symptoms of aging are mainly in the condition of the skin. It loses its youthful tight appearance and fresh color and becomes gray, dull, loose and flabby. Finally wrinkles appear all over, particularly on the face, neck and hands. These aging symptoms are largely due to the unhealthy state of collagen. Collagen is an elastic substance that holds all the tissues together—tissues of the muscles, organs, tendons, and last but not least, the tissues of the skin. When these connective tissues are healthy, they are strong and elastic and the skin is tight and has the look of youth. When collagen loses its tensile strength, muscles sag, the subcutaneous tissues (the layer just beneath the skin) become weak and lose their tension, and the skin becomes covered with wrinkles. What causes these degenerative changes in collagen? The answer is simple—the deficiency of vitamin C.

Now you can see why Russian scientists believe that they have found the Fountain of Youth in vitamin C.

Hardening of the arteries, atherosclerosis, and heart attacks are true diseases of premature aging. Many doctors believe that you are as old as your arteries. Recently, Boris Sokoloff, M.D., Director of the Southern Bio-Research Institute, Florida, reported that their conclusions, based on research and widespread evidence from medical literature, is that ascorbic acid (vitamin C) is the key factor in averting atherosclerosis, and that atherosclerosis (heart disease leading to heart attack) may, in fact, well be a vitamin C deficiency disease.[1]

The healthy function of sex glands is directly related to general health and to the prolonged feeling and appearance of youth. A Japanese doctor, M. Higuchi, has demonstrated that there is a relationship between vitamin C levels and the hormone production of the sex glands. In addition to vitamin C, vitamin E (which is sold in automatic dispensers in Sweden labeled as the sex-vitamin) plays an important part in the efficient activity of the sex glands. Prostatic fluid, which nourishes the sperm and keeps them alive, is extremely rich in vitamin C. A deficiency of vitamin C and vitamin E can slow down the hormone production of sex glands and consequently lead to premature aging.

Vitamin C—the miracle producer

If there ever has been a *real miracle drug,* vitamin C is it. It has so many universal applications that it is virtually impossible to find a condition of ill health, disease or diminished well-being which vitamin C would not affect favorably, very often with a miraculous healing effect. Since old age is often associated with various conditions of diminished health, it stands to reason that vitamin C should be a *rejuvenating tonic number one for everyone over 40 years of age.*

Do you get sufficient amounts of vitamin C in your diet? A recent Department of Agriculture report tells us that almost half of the American people eat diets deficient in vitamins C and A. Vitamin E is practically totally eliminated from American diet due to the refining of grains and oils; and available vitamin C in the American diet has been steadily declining for the last 20 years.

Swedish people have been using large amounts of vitamin C for centuries. Rose hips, the richest natural vitamin C source known to man (with the exception of acerola cherries), is a staple food in Sweden. They use it daily in the form of rose hip tea,* rose hip soup, rose hip puree*, etc.

Swedish people have another secret of staying young—whey. In Sweden whey is a staple food in the form of whey cheese and whey butter. In the United States you can obtain whey in a powder or tablet form from health food stores. Make a habit of eating some whey each day. It may surprise you by solving all your irregularity problems and make you feel—and look—ten years younger practically overnight!

REJUVENATION BULGARIAN STYLE

Ilja Metchnikoff, the famous Russian bacteriologist, revolutionized medical thinking on aging when he published his famous book *How to Prolong Life*. He advanced the theory that the secret of youth lies in the large intestine. He believed, and proved by experiments (as well as by long-living Bulgarians), that autotoxemia (selfpoisoning) through putrefaction of metabolic wastes in the large intestine is the main cause of premature aging. He was convinced

---

* See Chapter 16 for recipes and directions.

that if we could prevent the development of toxins in the colon, we could double the normal life span. Dr. Metchnikoff recommended the use of soured milk products, such as yogurt, kefir, acidophilus milk, etc., as a means of preventing putrefaction in the colon and bringing about the prolongation of life.

Bulgarians seem to be a living proof of Dr. Metchnikoff's theories. They live longer than most other people on earth and they also have comparatively more centenarians than any other country. It is well known that Bulgarians consume more soured milk in form of yogurt and kefir than any other nation.

There is extensive literature to support yogurt as a youthifying food. In order to prevent intestinal putrefaction and the consequent autointoxication, it is important to support and feed the friendly intestinal flora. This is best done with soured milk products and whey which contain lactose, the natural food for these bacteria.

Swedish Dr. E. M. Hoppe has made a very thorough study of Bulgarian centenarians and their living and eating habits. He made a detailed questioning of 158 Bulgarians of 100 years or older, and arrived at the following conclusions:

- Most of them were predominantly lacto-vegetarians: their diet consisted mainly of locally grown and stone ground whole grains, always freshly ground; fresh vegetables and fruits from their own gardens; and milk and milk products, predominantly from sheep milk. Only 5 of the 158 ate meat regularly.
- All of them ate yogurt, made mostly from sheep milk, regularly.
- Almost all of them were bee-keepers and used lots of honey in their diet.
- Almost all of them ate sunflower seeds regularly.
- They all ate fermented foods, especially sauerkraut.
- All have worked hard most of their lives, mostly on farms. Only 13 of the 158 lived most of their lives in cities.
- 110 of the 158 were extremely poor and could not afford to overeat.
- They were friendly, contented and had no great ambitions. They lived "without a clock," following nature's rhythm in sleeping, eating and working.

Here you have in a nutshell the Bulgarian secret of long, healthy life! No fancy secrets, tricky diets or drugs—just simple common-sense natural foods and wholesome, stress-free country life. But don't be deceived by its apparent simplicity: all the factors involved—a lacto-vegetarian diet of fresh vegetables and fruits, milk, yogurt, honey, sunflower seeds, fermented foods, and moderate eating—are scientifically proven as the most potent factors in preventing premature aging and prolonging life!

REJUVENATION RUMANIAN STYLE

Probably the most spectacular rejuvenation therapy of all times on a mass scale is the so-called *Gerovital* therapy. Gerovital is a *procaine* preparation, the rejuvenating effects of which were discovered by the Rumanian doctor, Professor Ana Aslan, M.D.

Professor Ana Aslan is very popular in Europe. Thousands upon thousands of people from all over the world travel to her Rejuvenation Institute in Bucharest and receive Gerovital treatments in hypermodern clinics under doctors' supervision. Dr. Aslan says that she has treated over 40,000 people in her Institute.

Dr. Aslan discovered quite accidently that procaine, previously commonly used as an anesthetic agent, had age-retarding property. She injected specially designed doses of *procaine,* which she named H_3, into patients showing signs of degeneration and premature aging, and observed that stiff, immobile joints became flexible, pain disappeared and the patients gained new energy and vitality. Dr. Aslan has improved her original H_3 formula and uses only Gerovital, which she claims has been demonstrated in tests in Italy and U.S.A. as being superior to pure procaine. Gerovital has been used in Rumania for 17 years, and presently 40,000 persons all over Rumania are under continuous prophylactic treatment with Gerovital. Dr. Aslan claims that Gerovital prolongs life and gives more energy, vitality and zest for living to older people. She recommends starting Gerovital treatments for preventive purposes at the age of 40. Between 40 and 60 Gerovital can be taken in tablet form. After 60, when absorbtion ability is diminished, she recommends injections.

According to Dr. Aslan, aging processes start when the body's ability to produce new cells and to replenish the old ones is diminished. Gerovital helps the body to regenerate new cell production, which is the reason for its rejuvenating effect.

I met Dr. Ana Aslan in Sweden, in the summer 1968, where she lectured on her rejuvenating method. She is a living advertisement for her drug and her therapy. At 72 she looks as though she is in her late fifties. Her face is quite free from wrinkles and even the skin on her arms is perfectly smooth and firm as on a younger person. I have also talked with several persons who undertook Gerovital therapy, and they all seemed to be enthusiastic about its revitalizing and rejuvenating effect.

Although Gerovital treatment is not endorsed by official medicine in most countries, it has an official sanction in Switzerland, Holland, Belgium, East Germany, and Rumania.

REJUVENATION RUSSIAN STYLE

The well-known Russian physiologist Tarkhanov wrote: "The time will come when it will be a disgrace for a man to die less than 100 years old."

There is extensive research going on in Russia on the prolongation of life. Russia is concentrating heavily on the preventive aspect of medicine. Russian medical scientists consider the prevention of disease and prolongation of life as their ultimate goals.

One of the Soviet scientists engaged in research on longevity is Dr. Olga Lepeshinskaya. In her book *Life, Age and Longevity,* she states that the *normal* life span of the human beings should be not less than *150 years,* if they would observe the elementary laws of health. Everyone who feels old before he reaches 100, she says, is suffering from *premature old age.* And she claims that premature old age, like other diseases, can be prevented; it also can be successfully treated after it appears. How? Her recipe is simple enough:

• sound, simple, natural nutrition;
• plenty of physical work, recreation and rest;
• a cheerful, optimistic outlook on life.

Here are some Russian longevity secrets, nutritionally speaking:

1. Food processing and refining is not as advanced in Russia as it is here; Russians still eat largely natural, unprocessed, unrefined foods.

2. There are very few additives allowed in food processing or manufacturing; all artificial colorings and flavorings are totally prohibited.

3. Russians eat very little meat compared to Americans. Only 25 percent of their protein intake is acquired from animal sources (in the United States it is 71 percent).

4. There are fewer devitalized foods and condiments available: no chewing gum, no Coca-Cola, no TV dinners.

Add to this less polluted water, virtually unpolluted air, no lead allowed in gasolines, more fertile soils, considerably less use of patented nonprescription drugs, and the great popularity of outdoor sports, hikes, bicycle tours, swimming, etc., and you can see why Russians are achieving better health and longer life. Their mortality rate is 7.6 per thousand against 9.4 in the United States and they have seven times more people reaching 100 years of age than has our country.

Here are a few other longevity points based on Russian medical discoveries and the experience of 21,000 Russian centenarians:

1. Russian scientists believe that vitamin C is the long-sought Fountain of Youth. They encourage Russians to collect wild rose hips and cultivate hip-bearing "vitamin roses" in their backyards for a plentiful supply of Vitamin C.

2. Russian scientists believe that vitamin E plays a vital role in staying younger longer and preventing premature aging. They prescribe vitamin E for the youthful function of sex glands and the healthy function of the reproductive system. At the Institute of Biochemistry of the Russian Academy of Science, experiments with vitamin E have shown that it has an emormously beneficial effect on the diseases of old age, specifically in combination with vitamin A. The rejuvenating property of these vitamins, aside from their direct effect on sex glands, is explained by the fact that they strengthen the ability of the tissues to absorb oxygen, restore impaired circulation in blood vessels, especially in the small capillaries, and help to restore the normal permeability of the blood vessels.

3. Studies of Russian centenarians show that almost all of them use lots of honey in their diet. Russian doctors encourage people to eat honey; they also prescribe honey as medicine and use it in hospitals, at bedtime, to induce a deep, restful sleep.

4. Russians eat enormous quantities of sunflower seeds and use unrefined cold-pressed sunflower oil. Sunflower oil is rich in vitamin E and essential fatty acids, the deficiency of which is definitely linked with premature aging. Sunflower seeds are also an excellent source of complete protein, B-vitamins, and minerals, especially *zinc,* which has been recently found to play an important role in the growth and maturity of the gonads, the sex glands, and is also directly linked with the health of the prostate gland. Zinc has been pointed out as an

active agent in most so-called virility foods, such as oysters, raw nuts, sea foods, onions, etc. Sunflower seeds and pumpkin seeds are very rich in this mineral.

5. Russians eat great amounts of raw onions and garlic, both considered by many nutritionists to be important life-prolongers.

6. Russian people eat lots of fermented foods; sour bread, sour pickles, sauerkraut, sour milk, kefir, yogurt. It has been demonstrated that fermented lactic-acid foods have an extremely cleansing and revitalizing effect on the digestive and assimilative tracts, and also have a direct curative effect, especially on the degenerative diseases. It could be, therefore, said that these foods have a rejuvenating effect.

THE SCIENCE OF MACROBIOTICS

A great physician, Christoph Wilhelm Hufeland, who lived in Berlin about 150 years ago, wrote a book to which he gave the title *Makrobiotik*—"The art of prolonging human life." Now, after 150 years, *macrobiotics* have become suddenly very popular in the United States. What are macrobiotics?

Hufeland's definition of macrobiotics was "the art of living longer." In the present technological and atomic age, macrobiotics means more than just "living longer." It is the study and application of fundamental factors essential for optimum health and longer life *free from disease*. Due to improved sanitation, reduction in infant mortality and modern surgery, man's average life expectancy has increased. But simultaneously, with the advance of technological and chemical sciences, the harmony between man and his natural health-giving environment has become disturbed. This disharmony has brought upon man a host of so-called degenerative diseases. Denatured, devitalized foods, a polluted and poisoned environment, the mental and physical stresses of the competitive world, have resulted in a gradual deterioration of health which has now reached catastrophic proportions.

It is hardly worthwhile to learn how to live a long life, if you have to live a life of miserable suffering from one agonizing disease after another. A long life would make sense only if it could be lived in vibrant health, enjoyed in the active productive pursuit of one's most treasured interests. The fact is that very few people now really enjoy perfect health. Most are sick, semi-ill or "fictitiously healthy," living in a chronic state of *mesotrophy,* or half-health.

Therefore, the modern meaning of macrobiotics is "the art of living longer in good health" or, in other words, *the art of living younger longer!*

I have referred previously to the International Society for Research on Nutrition and Vital Substances. The Scientific Counsel of this Society is composed of over 400 great scientists from 75 countries, representing doctors of medicine, bio-chemistry, nutrition, natural sciences, etc. A great many of these are Nobel Prize Winners. This most authoritative scientific forum conducts objective, scientific studies and research, and through its annual conventions disperses recommendations to various governments and their health organizations, as well as to the World Health Organization.

This Society has conducted a seven-year study of macrobiotics, or the fundamentals of healthier and longer life in our modern technological society. Its findings and conclusions in regard to macrobiotics were adopted at the Society's 7th International Convention.

Note this: you may read any number of popular health books or listen to the subjective, personal opinions of this or that health lecturer—usually with each one of them offering a different road to glorious health and long life—and you are no wiser in the end. But here is the united consensus of a large body of responsible and respected scientists, based on the objective study and research of all available scientific data. It would be wise to listen to them.

The following résumé is based on Resolution No. 25 of the International Society for Research on Nutrition and Vital Substances.

Civilization's diseases and their basic causes

Civilization, increased industrialization and artificial, altered environment have caused a dangerous increase in various diseases, which are called civilization diseases. These are: dental diseases, chronic stomach and intestinal diseases, heart and coronary diseases, rheumatic diseases, some nervous disorders, and cancer.

The basic causes of civilization diseases are to be found in our antibiological way of living, such as:

• Changes in environment: air and water pollution, etc.

- Changes in nutrition: health-destroying toxic food additives, foods grown in depleted soils and devitalized by processing, wrong selection of diet, overeating, etc.
- Disturbances of life rhythm: lack of exercise, haste and hurry, insufficient rest and recreation, excessive use of tobacco, alcohol, and drugs, etc.

Civilization diseases can be cured or prevented, and a long life in good health can be accomplished, by the following remedial measures:

1. Improved nutrition from natural unadulterated foods, free from toxic additives and rich in vital substances (enzymes, vitamins, minerals, trace elements, proteins, etc.).

2. Intensified battle against the continuous pollution of water, air, soil, and food, which causes the accumulation of toxic substances in our bodies, and ultimately disease.

3. Improved safety and hygenic conditions at work.

4. Sufficient recreation and rest.

Points 2, 3, and 4 are self-explanatory. In regard to point No. 1, *improved nutrition,* the Society gives the following advice:

The basis of a diet which assures healthy and well-balanced nutrition should be:

- *Cereal products:* whole grain cereals and breads, and other courses from whole corn, whole rice, and other whole grains and seeds.
- *Milk and milk products:* cheese, curds (cottage cheese), soured milk, yogurt, kefir and butter (moderately). Milk and milk products should *not* be pasteurized.
- *Vegetables, fruits, and potatoes.* Fruits and vegetables preferably should be consumed *raw;* potatoes peeled after cooking.

In addition, the following recommendations are given:

- *Meat, fish and eggs* can supplement this basic diet, but a daily intake of these foods is *not necessary.*
- *Unrefined, cold-pressed vegetable oils,* rich in unsaturated fatty acids, such as sunflower oil, linseed oil, soybean oil, should be included in the diet.
- *Honey* should replace the use of white sugar and sweets.
- The fact that about half of the world population lives on a vegetable diet proves the possibility of *vegetarian nutrition.*
- In order to assure complete nutritional balance, a vegetarian diet should be supplemented with milk and milk products,

nuts, soybeans, linseed, sunflower seeds, edible yeast, fruit juices, etc.

- Older persons should increase intake of *honey* and *vitamins; avoid overeating,* especially of *animal fats;* and *restrict salt* intake.
- All foods should be as natural as possible, without chemical additives.

So, here you have, *from the highest possible authoritative source on nutrition, a macrobiotic diet which will assure you optimal health and prolong your life.*

HEALTH, LONG LIFE AND SEXUAL VIRILITY

The Russian Minister of Health told the story of a Russian centenarian from Caucasus who lived to the respectable age of 146 years. When asked for the reasons for his enviable longevity, the man said:

"I have never had a boss over me—I have never been envious of what others have—and I have periodically rejuvenated myself by marrying three times!"

Vibrant health, long life and sexual virility go hand in hand. All vital functions of the body should collaborate in perfect harmony, including the functions of the vital reproductive system. The health of the reproductive system is closely tied to the general state of health, which is, as we have already seen, dependent on vital nutrition.

In the last ten years many studies have been made which indicate that man's sexuality is not an isolated phenomenon, but is an inseparable part of his total health entity. Doctors have found that man's sexual capacity is directly related to his health and his mental and physical well-being. Furthermore, they have found that there is a direct relationship between man's sexual health and the foods he eats. Recognizing that psychological causes are behind many cases of impotency and other sexual disturbances, the fact remains that nutrition is the most important single factor affecting one's health, including the health of the reproductive system. Malnutrition and nutritional deficiencies may affect every aspect of man's physical well-being. His sexual functions are no exception.

Just how does nutrition affect man's sex life?

Man's sexual life is directed by his glandular system, particularly by the so-called endocrine glands. The hormones produced by these glands, and by the ovaries and testes, hold the secret of your sexual power. *Estrogen* plays a vital part in the sexual life and reproductive functions of women; *testosterone,* the male sex hormone, plays an equally important part in man's sexual life. These hormones and other secretions of the endocrine glands are your spark plugs, which provide sex stimulus and drive to your body as well as to your mind. The decreased function of the endocrine glands and diminished secretion of sex hormones will slow down all vital life processes and lead to premature aging. The healthy function of the endocrine glands is imperative not only for sexual virility and libido, but is also absolutely essential for your general health and for your feeling and looking younger far into advanced age. In other words, you are as old as your glands!

What can you do to keep your endocrine and sex glands in good working condition so that you will remain vital and virile as long as you live?

You can feed your glands! Your glands need certain nutrients in order to function properly. If the food you eat does not supply these essential nutrients, the normal function of the glands will be impaired, and hormone production diminished. Lost interest in sex and diminished or totally lost physical capacity for love will be the ultimate result.

Since the beginning of time man had certain remedies and foods for prolonging or increasing his sexual power. Every nation and every race had their favorites: honey, sesame seeds, oysters, nuts, eggs, etc. Modern medical science laughed at the notion that there is a relationship between food and man's physical capacity for love. But in the last decade or two we have seen profound changes taking place in the attitudes of scientists toward sex. Doctors stopped laughing and began a serious inquiry into the mysteries of sex life. Now it is not only an old wives' tale, but a well-established scientific fact that your libido and capacity for physical love are directly related to your nutrition.

It would take a book to relate to you all the exciting facts the scientists are coming up with with regard to the relationship between nutrition and sex. Much research is being done in Russia, France, and Germany in this field. There is also corroborative research being done in the United States. Here are a few revealing facts discovered by scientists.

1. Zinc

Several studies indicate that a deficiency of the trace mineral zinc may be associated with poor sexual performance due to retarded genital development or hypogonadism. Medical researchers have found that in Iran and Egypt, where many people live on zinc-deficient diets, many boys suffer from the retarded development and growth of the gonads—the sex organs. When the diet is supplemented with zinc, they rapidly mature sexually.

Zinc has also been found to play a vital role in the health of the prostate. There is a very high concentration of zinc in the sperm, the seminal fluid, and in the prostate itself—more than in any other part of the body. A deficiency of zinc causes enlargement of the prostate and other unhealthy changes in this vital sex gland. Thus, zinc is definitely related to man's sexual performance and potential. This is especially important to men past middle age, when prostate troubles usually start.

Is it possible to have deficiency of zinc if you eat a normal well-balanced diet? Yes, more likely than not, your diet is deficient in it. First, the soil of 32 of our 50 states is deficient in zinc, and the nutritive elements in your food can come only from the soil. Then, zinc is taken out of our foods by refining and processing, especially when bran and germ are removed from the grains. Foods rich in zinc are oysters (long believed by folklore to be a source of virility), herring, wheat bran and wheat germ, brewer's yeast, onions, and eggs. Sunflower and pumpkin seeds are an excellent source of zinc, also.

2. Pumpkin seeds

A German doctor has discovered that in certain countries, where pumpkin seeds are eaten regularly and in great quantity, there is virtually no incidence of enlarged prostate or other prostate troubles. Dr. W. Devrient states that enlargement of the prostate gland indicates that the gland is trying to make up for the diminished production of the male sex hormones as a result of advanced age. Pumpkin seeds contain nutrients which are essential for reproductive functions.

Pumpkin seeds are extremely rich in powerful nutritive factors: about 30 percent protein, 40 percent unsaturated fatty acids, plenty of B-vitamins, lots of phosphorus, iron, and *zinc*. What is the powerful substance in pumpkin seed that has such a rejuvenating effect on sex life? No one seems to know. Dr. Bela Pater, of Klausenburg, believes that pumpkin seeds contain a "plant hormone which affects man's hormone production in part by substitution, in part by direct proliferation." But whatever substance it is, the fact remains that, as of today, pumpkin seeds are the only effective nutritional remedy for prostate trouble—and completely harmless, too.

3. Vitamin E and wheat germ oil

A friend of mine in Canada, Mrs. K., had seven early miscarriages during eight years of marriage. She was unimpressed by my repeated advice to try wheat germ oil and vitamin E, because her obstetrician didn't think it was worth considering. However, when another friend, a veterinarian, told her that this was exactly the treatment he had been using successfully on horses and cows with records of miscarriage, she decided to try. Within three months she became pregnant and, after a full nine-month pregnancy, delivered a healthy boy.

The healthy functioning of the reproductive system is dependent on many factors. Both psychological and physiological causes must be considered. Nutrition is, of course, a most vital factor. Many vitamins and other nutritive substances are directly involved in a healthy sex life. But if there was one vitamin which could be called the *sex vitamin,* then it would be vitamin E.

It has been established that vitamin E can prevent miscarriage and stillbirths. Vitamin E is essential for the normal production of sex hormones. It has been demonstrated in animal tests that when vitamin E is deficient, the testicles degenerate and production of hormones is diminished—both sex hormones and pituitary hormones, which stimulate sex glands.[2] Vitamin E, being a natural and powerful anti-oxidant, also protects sex hormones from destruction by oxidation. Dr. Evan Shute of Canada, a pioneer in the use of vitamin E for disorders in the reproductive system, has used vitamin E extensively and successfully in the treatment of various disorders from male sterility to miscarriages and menopausal symptoms. In one study he used vitamin E in 153 pregnancies in which there were 122 threatened abortions and 87 threatened miscarriages. 60 percent of the abortions and 86 percent of the miscarriages were prevented by vitamin E treatment. Dr. Shute says that vitamin E deficiency is very common in pregnant women.

Vitamin E has also been found to relieve the symptoms of menopause, or change of life: hot flashes, dizziness, pain, etc. Doses of 150 to 300 milligrams a day are prescribed in such cases. A Hungarian doctor has found that vitamin E decreases pain in childbirth labor.

Vitamin E is, indeed, absolutely essential for the normal function of the reproductive system and a healthy sex life. The best natural source of vitamin E is wheat germ oil and wheat germ. Other good sources are cold-pressed vegetable oils, such as corn oil, soybean oil, and sunflower seed oil. Green vegetables are also good sources, particularly cauliflower, turnips, and spinach. Milk and dairy products are also good sources. You can also buy vitamin E in capsule form at health food stores or drug stores. Doses most often recommended by doctors are between 300 and 600 I.U. per day.

4. Milk

Milk, especially goat milk, has been held in high repute, especially in Hindu countries, as a potent virility food. The exceptional property of milk is explained by the fact that protein is an extremely important nutrient for normal sex functions. Milk protein, casein, is the highest grade of protein known to man. Furthermore, milk proteins are very easily digested and more fully utilized than any other form of protein. The combination of "milk and honey" is a simple but powerful evening drink to combat "bedroom fatigue." Note that milk also contains vitamin B_{12}. Adelle Davis relates in her excellent book *Let's Get Well* the case of a couple who had lost all interest in sex, but recaptured it again after eating a diet she prescribed for their son; the diet specified increased milk intake and the addition of wheat germ and yeast. The woman told Adelle Davis that this diet had saved her marriage and was largely responsible for their revitalized sex life.

5. Sesame seeds

In Chapter 16 you will find a recipe for homemade halvah. Halvah is made from sesame seeds and honey. It has been used in the Orient for thousands of years as a popular candy. Even now, halvah is very popular in the Middle East—in Turkey, Israel, and the Arabian countries. In ancient Babylon women ate halvah to restore their vitality and sex appeal.

A French doctor's research a few years ago gave scientific support to the old folklore. Sesame seeds have been found to be rich in the minerals magnesium and potassium, and honey is rich in aspartic acid, one of the amino acids. A New Jersey doctor has used very similar ingredients in a prescription drug to treat hundreds of women with what he calls "the housewife syndrome," or chronic fatigue, insomnia and lethargy in lovemaking. 87 percent of his patients responded with a startling change in their condition: their fatigue and lethargy disappeared and they became cheerful and energetic.

Sesame seeds are one of the real wonder foods of nature. They are extremely rich in calcium; in fact they are richer in calcium than milk, cheese or nuts. Their protein content is high, too—19 to 28 percent—higher than meats; and sesame protein is of a very high quality. Sesame seeds are also very rich in unsaturated fatty acids and lecithin, in B-vitamins, especially inositol and choline, and they also are a good source of vitamin E—all substances vital for the health of the reproductive system.

Sesame is one of the earliest grains cultivated by man. Even now in many countries of the East, Middle East and East Europe, sesame seeds are a staple food. In the United States, you can buy plain sesame seeds or many various products made from sesame in health food stores. There is halvah, sesame seed oil, and many kinds of peanut-butter-like spreads.

YOU ARE AS YOUNG AS YOUR NUTRITION

All in all, you can see that *the secret of staying young is basically the secret of staying healthy*. And the secret of staying healthy is closely tied to proper nutrition. More and more researchers of the noble science of Gerontology come, in their quest for the secrets of aging, to the inevitable conclusion that the Fountain of Youth springs from *vital nutrition*.

It could be truthfully said that:
- you are as young as your glands;
- you are as young as your cells;
- you are as young as your collagen;
- you are as young as your enzymes and your digestive system;
- you are as young as your arteries and your heart.

But in order to keep your glands and organs young, your colon free from decay and putrifaction, your collagen elastic and your cells healthy and vital, you have to feed your body with the highest quality vital nutrition, which contains all the essential nutrients necessary for the normal function of all these organs and tissues.

Of course, the state of your mind has a determining influence on your health, too. But even the state of your mind, your attitudes, your mental capacities—yes, even the strength of your moral fiber—all depend to a great extent on the quality of your nutrition. *"Mens sana in corpore sano"* said the old Romans, and this is just as true today. A sound mind can only dwell in a sound body.

The more we search for the secrets of aging the more we become convinced that you cannot discuss the problems of premature aging without discussing the problems of nutrition.

Dr. Henry C. Sherman of Columbia University, one of the greatest authorities on nutrition, has stated that not only can human life be extended, but also youthfulness can be preserved and the extended life span made more useful, by the right selection of foods.

Recently, the Journal of the American Geriatrics Society reported on research by a Hungarian scientist, who has found that malnutrition is a prime cause of premature aging.

HOW TO PREVENT PREMATURE AGING AND STAY YOUNGER LONGER

Which foods will give you longer life and keep you younger longer? The macrobiotic diet outlined in this chapter will improve your health and increase your longevity. It is a predominantly lacto-vegetarian diet high in *natural* carbohydrates and low in animal proteins. The bulk of this diet consists of raw fruits and vegetables, whole grain products, milk and milk products, plus seeds, nuts, honey and vegetable oils. Meat, fish and eggs should be excluded totally or used in moderation—fish and eggs used in preference to meat. Remember, the healthiest peoples in the world, known for their longevity, who live in Bulgaria, Russia and Hunza, eat very little meat; and a surprisingly high percentage of Russian and Bulgarian centenarians are vegetarians.

Here are a few other important longevity points to remember:

1. Get plenty of physical excercise, avoid mental and emotional stresses, and get sufficient sleep and relaxation.

2. Supplement your diet with such natural nutritional substances as brewer's or food yeast, kelp, cod liver oil (in winter months) and rose hips and whey—all potent longevity foods.

3. Avoid: white sugar, white flour, coffee, tea, tobacco, salt, canned, preserved and irradiated foods, processed cereals, all refined and adulterated foods.

4. Make an effort to obtain organically grown foods, raised without chemical fertilizers and poisonous pesticides.

5. Soured milk in the form of yogurt,* buttermilk or kefir* are longevity foods because of their beneficial effect on the intestinal tract. Also other fermented lactic-acid foods, such as sauerkraut,* sour pickles,* and sour-dough bread,* are established macrobiotic factors. Use them liberally.

6. It has been established that an active sex life is tied to overall good health and longevity. A healthy hormone-producing activity of the endocrine glands and the sex glands has a powerful influence on the health, and consequently is an important factor for potential longevity. An atrophied glandular system and diminished hormone production bring about premature aging and senility. The following foods have been found to have a beneficial protective and stimulating effect on the normal functions of the glandular and reproductive systems:

- wheat germ oil and wheat germ;
- sesame seeds, sunflower seeds, and pumpkin seeds;
- honey—raw, unrefined, unheated;
- milk and cheese—raw, unpasteurized, unprocessed;
- brewer's yeast or food yeast.

Follow the macrobiotic diet outlined in this chapter and adhere to the advice in the above six points and you can assure yourself of the best possible health throughout your life. At the same time, this macrobiotic program will prevent premature aging, give you longer life and keep you young longer. This program is in harmony with the recomendations by the most authoritative scientific forum: the International Society for Research on Nutrition and Vital Substances. And, if my own humble opinion is of any value to you, I can testify—after giving this rejuvenating macrobiotic system a 20-year try—that it definitely "works"!

---

* See Chapter 16 for recipe and directions.

16

Recipes and Directions for Special European Health and Longevity Foods

Below are recipes and directions for preparing cereals, salads, breads, and other health and longevity foods named and recommended in this book. Most of the ingredients mentioned in the recipes are available at better health food stores.

BIRCHER-BENNER APPLE MÜESLI

2 tbsp. old-fashioned rolled oats (not the quick-cooking kind)
2 medium-sized apples
2 tbsp. wheat germ
2 tbsp. condensed milk or ordinary milk, fortified with 1 tbsp. skim milk powder
2 tbsp. honey
½ lemon
2 tbsp. chopped hazel nuts or almonds

Soak oatmeal overnight in four tablespoons of water. In the morning, add lemon juice and milk; mix well. Shred apples, unpeeled but well washed, into the mixture. Add honey, wheat germ and nuts, and stir. Serve at once, as it will lose in taste and food value if apples darken (oxidize) .

This dish is a favorite at the famous Bircher-Benner biological clinic in Switzerland and is also very popular in health food restaurants in Europe.

FRUIT SALAD À LA AIROLA

> 1 bowl fresh fruits, organically grown if possible
> 1 handful raw nuts and/or sunflower seeds
> 3–4 soaked prunes or handful of raisins, unsulphured
> 3 tbsp. cottage cheese, preferably homemade, unsalted
> 1 tbsp. raw wheat germ
> 1 tsp. wheat germ oil
> 3 tbsp. yogurt
> 2 tsp. natural, unpasteurized honey
> 1 tsp. fresh lemon juice

Wash all fruits carefully and dry. Use any available fruits and berries, but try to get at least three or four different kinds. Peaches, grapes, pears, papaya, bananas, and fresh pineapple are particularly good for producing a delightful bouquet of rich, penetrating flavors. A variety of colors will make the salad festive and attractive to the eye.

Chop or slice bigger fruits, but leave grapes and berries whole. Place them in a large bowl and add prunes and nuts (nuts and sunflower seeds could be crushed) . Make a dressing with one teaspoon of honey (or more if most of the fruits used are sour) , one teaspoon of lemon juice, and two tablespoons of water. Pour over the fruit, add wheat germ, and toss well. Mix cottage cheese, yogurt, wheat germ oil, and one teaspoon of honey in a separate cup until it is fairly smooth in texture and pour it on top of the salad. Sprinkle with nuts and sunflower seeds. Serve at once.

This is not only a most delicious dish but it is the most nutritious and perfectly balanced meal I know. It is a storehouse of high-grade proteins and all the essential vitamins, minerals, and enzymes you need for optimum health. This salad should be a daily *must* for the beauty-conscious and health-conscious alike.

WAERLAND FIVE-GRAIN KRUSKA

(for 4 persons)

1 tbsp. whole wheat
1 tbsp. whole rye
1 tbsp. whole oats
1 tbsp. whole barley
1 tbsp. whole millet
2 tbsp. wheat bran
2 tbsp. unsulphured raisins

Take five grains and grind them coarsely on your own grinder. Place in a pot with one to one and a half cups of water and add bran and raisins. Boil for five to ten minutes, then wrap the pot in a blanket or newspapers and let it stand for a few hours. Experiment with the amount of water used—kruska must not be mushy, but should have the consistency of a very thick porridge. Serve hot with sweet milk and homemade applesauce or stewed fruits.

Kruska is an extremely nutritious dish and should be taken as a meal in itself.

UNCOOKED QUICK KRUSKA

Use the same ingredients as above. Pour boiling water over freshly ground grains and other ingredients and let stand and steep for about half an hour. This Quick Kruska is delicious and more easily digestible because of the preserved enzymes. Serve warm and eat the same way as the cooked Five-grain Kruska.

HOMEMADE APPLESAUCE

Use only unsprayed apples. Sprayed apples should be carefully brushed and washed or peeled. Cut up whole apples—peel, core and all—and stew in a small quantity of water until soft. Use a stainless steel utensil and only enough water to cover the bottom. Sweeten with honey, if necessary. If the apples are sweet, no sweetening is needed. When apples are soft, pass them through a sieve or blend in a blender. Keep in refrigerator.

KASHA (buckwheat cereal)

1 cup whole buckwheat grains
2 cups water

Bring water to a boil. Stir the buckwheat into the boiling water and let boil for two to three minutes. Turn heat to low and simmer for 15 to 20 minutes, stirring occasionally. If seasoning is desired use a very little sea salt. When all the water is absorbed, take from the stove and let stand for another 15 minutes. Kasha must never be mushy. Serve hot with sunflower seed oil or butter.

This is a favorite cereal in Russia and many other Eastern European countries. It has an unusual mellow flavor and it is extremely nutritious.

MILLET CEREAL

1 cup hulled millet
3 cups water
½ tsp. honey
½ cup powdered skim milk

Rinse millet in warm water and drain. Place in a pan of water mixed with powdered skim milk and heat mixture to boiling point. Then simmer for ten minutes, stirring occasionally to prevent sticking and burning. Remove from heat and let stand for a half hour or more. Serve with milk, honey, oil, or butter—or homemade applesauce! And treat yourself to the *most nutritious cereal in the world!*

Note: when you buy millet see that it has a bright yellow color. When millet gets old it changes color from bright yellow to a light gray or dull grayish-yellow.

MOLINO CEREAL

1 tbsp. coarse whole wheat flour
2 tbsp. wheat bran
2 tbsp. whole flaxseed

2–3 chopped figs or soaked prunes, or
1 tbsp. unsulphured raisins

Place all the ingredients in a pan with one cup of water and boil for five minutes, stirring occasionally to prevent burning. Serve immediately with sweet milk, a little honey, or homemade applesauce.

This cereal is served in European clinics to patients with weak digestion and a tendency toward constipation.

POTATO CEREAL

2 large raw potatoes
2 tbsp. whole wheat flour
1 tbsp. wheat bran
1 tbsp. wheat germ
4 cups water

Heat water to boiling point. Mix flour and bran in pan and simmer for two to three minutes. Place a fine shredder over pan and quickly shred potatoes directly into pan. Stir vigorously and lift from the stove. Let stand for a few minutes and serve hot with milk, butter, or cream; sprinkle wheat germ on top.

This is an alkaline and exceptionally nutritious cereal. It is used often in Swedish biological clinics, especially in diets for patients with rheumatic diseases.

SPROUTED WHEAT

There are many different methods of sprouting seeds. Waerland recommends the following method: soak the wheat grains in water at room temperature for three nights and spread them thinly on a dish or paper towel for three days. To prevent the grains from molding they must be rinsed under running water three times a day. When the sprouts are the length of the seed they are ready for eating.

Another good method is to soak wheat overnight in cold water, then roll the scattered seeds inside a wet clean towel. Sprinkle water over the towel several times a day.

In the treatment of multiple sclerosis one or two tablespoons of sprouted wheat is given daily. Sprouted beans and seeds are excellent health foods, and everyone can benefit by using them regularly.

HALVAH

1 cup sesame seeds
2 tsp. honey, preferably coagulated solid honey

Grind sesame seeds on a small electric seed grinder. Pour sesame meal into a larger cup and knead honey into the meal with a large spoon until honey is well mixed and the halvah acquires the consistency of a hard dough. Serve it as it is, or make small balls and roll them in whole sesame seeds, shredded coconut, or sunflower seeds.

HOMEMADE SOURED MILK

Use only unpasteurized, raw milk. Place a bottle of milk in a pan filled with warm water and warm it to about body temperature. Fill a cup or a deep plate, stir in tablespoon of yogurt, cover with paper towel (for dust) and keep in warm place—for example, near the stove, heating radiator, or wherever there is a constant warm temperature. The milk will coagulate in approximately 24 hours.

Use one or two spoonfuls of soured milk as a culture for your next batch (use yogurt or commercial buttermilk only as a starting culture for the first batch) .

HOMEMADE COTTAGE CHEESE

Take homemade soured milk and warm it to about 140° F—but not higher than 160° F (70° C) —by placing the container in warm water. When the milk has curdled, place a clean linen canvas over a deep strainer and pour curdled milk over it. Wait until all liquid whey has seeped through the strainer. What remains in the strainer is fresh, wholesome, and delicious homemade cottage cheese. If the cheese is too hard, add a little sweet or sour cream, and stir. The higher the temperature the harder the cheese, and vice versa.

By the way, don't throw the whey away—it is an exceptionally nutritious, beautifying and rejuvenating drink.

HOMEMADE YOGURT

Take a bottle of skim milk and heat it until it almost, but not quite, boils. Add two to three tablespoons of yogurt, which can be bought in a grocery store or health shop. Stir well. Pour into a wide-mouthed thermos bottle. Cover and let it stand overnight. In five to eight hours it will be solid and ready to serve. If you do not have a thermos jar, use an ordinary glass jar and place it in a pan of warm water over an electric burner switched on "warm" for four to five hours, then switch off until milk is solid.

Use two to three spoonfuls of your fresh, homemade yogurt as a culture for the next batch.

HOMEMADE KEFIR

To make your own kefir you will need kefir grains. There is a mail order company, R. A. J. Biological Laboratory, 35 Park Avenue, Blue Point, Long Island, N.Y. which sells kefir grains by mail directly to customers. The price is between $5.00 and $10.00 postpaid for a unit. The kefir grains will last indefinitely; there is never any need to reorder. Merely follow the instructions which will come with each order.

Place 1 tbsp. of kefir grains in a glass of milk, stir and allow to stand at room temperature overnight. When the milk coagulates it is ready for eating. Kefir is a true "elixir of youth," used by centenarians in Bulgaria, Russia and Caucasus as a part of their daily diet.

VEGETABLE BROTH

2 large potatoes, chopped or sliced to approximately half-inch pieces
1 cup carrots, shredded or sliced
1 cup celery, chopped or shredded, leaves and all
1 cup any other available vegetable: beet tops, turnip tops, parsley, or a little of everything. (However, broth can be made with only potatoes, carrots, and celery.)

Put all vegetables into a stainless steel utensil, add one and a half quarts of water, cover and cook slowly for about a half-hour. Strain, cool until warm, and serve. If not used immediately keep in refrigerator and warm up before serving.

Vegetable broth is one of the standard beverages in all biological clinics in Sweden. Fasting patients always start the day with a big mug of vegetable broth, a cleansing and alkalizing, mineral-rich drink.

EXCELSIOR

    1 cup of vegetable broth, as above
    1 tbsp. whole flaxseed
    1 tbsp. wheat bran

Soak flaxseed and wheat bran in vegetable broth overnight. In the morning, warm up, stir well, and drink—seeds and all. Do not chew the flaxseeds, drink them whole. Excelsior drink is especially beneficial for patients with constipation problems. It helps to restore normal peristaltic rhythm. When used during fasting Excelsior must be strained.

ROSE HIP TEA

Take one tablespoon of dried rose hips or rose hip powder for each cup of water. Bring to a boil, but do not actually boil, then steep for five minutes (for powder) or 15 minutes (for whole or halves). Strain, sweeten with honey, and enjoy a vitamin C-loaded, nutritious and beautifying pink-colored tea. Imported Scandinavian rose hips and rose hip powder can be bought in health food stores, even in the United States.

Note: do not use aluminum utensils when cooking rose hips.

SWEDISH ROSE HIP SOUP

Take two tablespoons of rose hip powder for each cup of water or for each serving. Boil in pan for five minutes. Sweeten with honey and thicken with a half-tablespoon of corn starch or potato flour per serving. Soybean flour can also be used to make the soup even more nutritious. After adding the thickening, boil again for three minutes.

Serve warm or chilled. Can be served with sweet milk or cream, and sprinkled with wheat germ, crushed raw nuts, or sunflower seeds. An excellent, beautifying dessert!

ROSE HIP PURÉE

If you can gather your own rose hips in the fall, here's how you can make rose hip puree from fresh rose hips.

Remove the stalks and the blossom ends of the berries. Cut or break berries in half and remove the seeds and the "hair" from the shells with your fingers. Take one pound of rose hips for each pint of water. Bring to a boil and simmer for about 10 to 15 minutes. Then press through a sieve, or mix in a blender. Serve hot or cold. Sweeten with honey.

SOUR RYE BREAD
(Black Bread Russian Style)

8 cups freshly ground whole rye flour
3 cups warm water
½ cup sourdough culture

Mix seven cups of flour with water and sourdough culture. Cover and let stand in a warm place overnight between 12 and 18 hours. Add remaining flour and mix well. Place in greased pans. Let it rise for approximately a half-hour. Bake at 350° F, one hour or more, if needed. Always save a half-cup of dough as a culture for the next baking. Keep the culture in a tight jar in your refrigerator. For the initial baking it will be necessary to obtain a sourdough culture from a commercial bakery.

This recipe makes two two-pound loaves.

HOMEMADE SAUERKRAUT

Use a small wooden barrel, or a large earthenware pot. Possibly a large stainless steel pail or a glass jar could be used, but under no circumstances use an aluminum utensil.

Cut white cabbage heads into narrow strips with a large knife or grater, and place in a barrel. When the layer of cabbage is about four to six inches deep, sprinkle a few juniper berries, cummin seeds and/or black currant leaves on top—use your favorite or whatever you have available. A few strips of carrots, green peppers, and onions can also be used. Add a little sea salt—not more than two ounces for each 25 pounds of cabbage. Then add another layer of grated cabbage and spices until the container is filled. Each layer should be pressed and stamped very hard with your fists or a piece of wood so that there will be no air left and the cabbage will be saturated with its own juice.

When the container is full, cover cabbage with a clean linen canvas, place a wooden or slate board over it, and on the top place a clean heavy stone. Let stand for three to four weeks in a warm place, not below 70° F. Now and then remove the foam and the possible mildew from the top, from the stone and from the barrel edges. The linen canvas, board and stone should be occasionally removed, washed well with warm and then cold water, and replaced. After three to four weeks the sauerkraut is ready for eating. It can be left in the barrel, which now should be stored in a cool place, or put in glass jars and kept in the refrigerator.

Sauerkraut is best eaten *raw*—both from the point of taste and for its health-giving value. Drink sauerkraut juice, too. It is an extremely beneficial and wonderfully nutritious drink.

HOMEMADE SOUR PICKLES

Use only small, fresh, hard cucumbers. Place them in cold water overnight, then dry them well.

Place cucumbers in a wooden barrel, or a large earthenware or glass jar. Place a few leaves of black currants, cherries, mustard seed and dill branches in with the cucumbers.

Boil up a sufficient amount of salt water, using about four ounces of sea salt for five quarts of water. Let water cool down, then pour it over cucumbers. Cover with linen canvas, place a wooden board over it, and on the top a clean heavy stone. There should be enough salt water to cover the board. Keep container in a warm place for about one week, then move to a cooler place. Pickles are ready for eating in about three to four weeks. Every second week or so remove the stone and the covers and wash them well first in warm then in cold water, then replace them. Keep the top of the water clean from foam and mildew. When pickles are ready for eating they can be placed in glass jars and kept in the refrigerator.

Epilogue

There are hundreds of clinics in Europe, especially in Germany, Sweden, and Switzerland, where the biological therapies described in this book are applied. If you have an opportunity to travel to Europe and wish to visit some of these clinics, you can find their names and addresses in health magazines available in most European health food stores.

Of course, many of the do-it-yourself treatments and dietary programs recommended in this book, including juice fasting, can be safely undertaken on your own. However, if you suffer from a serious illness, such as a severe heart condition, extremely high blood pressure, diabetes, etc., my advice is to consult your doctor, show him this book and the therapies described, and follow his advice in regard to the advisability of undertaking a program of biological treatment in your case. If your doctor is reluctant to try biological therapy, find another doctor, who is more openminded, unprejudiced, and bio-logically- (and nutritionally-) oriented. Naturopathic and osteo-pathic physicians are generally sympathetic toward biological thera-pies. There are also many medical doctors in this country who are well informed on biological medicine and find nothing objectionable in the programs outlined in this book. Perhaps your health food store or the local chapter of the National Health Federation can recom-mend such a doctor. Or write to me in care of the Parker Publishing Company, West Nyack, N.Y., enclosing a self-addressed envelope. I may be able to advise on doctors or clinics in the United States, Mexico and Canada specializing in the biological therapies recom-mended in this book; since the 1968 publication of my book *There Is a Cure for Arthritis*, several doctors have written to me telling of their successful experiences with biological therapies.

Doctors who desire to investigate in more detail the treatments outlined in this book should study the sources of research and information given in the references. Also, I urge doctors to subscribe to the following most reliable and abundant source of information on proven biological medical treatments for various diseases: *Biologisch Medizinisches Taschen Jahrbuch,* Hippokrates Verlag, GmbH. Stuttgart, West Germany. This informative yearly book (in the German language) is used by thousands of medical doctors in Germany and other countries.

ACKNOWLEDGMENTS

I wish to express my sincere thanks and indebtedness to the editors of the Swedish magazine *Tidskrift För Hälsa,* Eskil Svensson and Arne Algard, for their cooperation and kindness in granting me permission to use material from the magazine. Chapters 2, 7, 9, and 14 are in part based on the articles published in *Tidskrift För Hälsa.*

I am particularly indebted to Dr. Jern Hamberg, for proof-reading the manuscript and for his valuable advice which resulted in many pertinent changes in the contents of this book.

Footnote References
Keyed to Chapters

Chapter 1

[1] *Journal of the American Dietetic Association,* January, 1967.
[2] *Journal of the American Medical Association,* February 21, 1966.
[3] *Public Health Service Annual Supplement,* Vol. 8, No. 53, September 16, 1960.

Chapter 2

[1] Paavo O. Airola, *There Is a Cure for Arthritis,* Parker Publishing Company, Inc., West Nyack, N.Y., 1968.
[2] Arnold DeVries, *Therapeutic Fasting,* Chandler Book Co., Los Angeles, 1963.

Chapter 3

[1] Ruth Bircher, *Eating Your Way to Health,* Faber and Faber, London.

Chapter 4

[1] *Current Therapeutic Research,* March, 1961.
[2] *Some New Aspects of Spa Therapy in Rheumatology,* a release from the Hungarian Legation in London, England.
[3] T. Hartley-Hennessy, A.R.C.A., *Healing by Water,* C. W. Daniel Co., England.

Chapter 5

[1] Are and Ebba Waerland, *Health Is Your Birthright,* Humata Publishers, Bern, Switzerland.

Chapter 6

[1] Prof. H. A. Schweigart, *Eiweiss, Fette, Herzinfarkt,* Verlag H. H. Zauner, Munchen.

[2] Prof. Karl Eimer (Klinik Schwenkenbacker), *Zeitschrift für Ernahrung,* July, 1933.

[3] *Dr. Bircher-Benner's Way to Positive Health and Vitality,* Bircher-Benner Verlag, Zürich, Switzerland.

[4] *Resolution No. 80,* International Society for Research on Nutrition and Vital Substances.

[5] "Nutritional Contributions of Wheat," *The Journal of the American Medical Association,* November 29, 1948.

[6] *Tidskrift För Hälsa,* November, 1967.

[7] Dr. Ralph Bircher, "Raw Food—A Potent Factor in Acquiring Positive Health," from the address in Sidney, Australia, October 26, 1967.

[8] L. T. Miller, *et al., Journal of Nutrition,* September, 1967.

[9] *A.M.A. News Release,* June 21, 1965.

[10] *New York Times,* April 7, 1965.

[11] W. A. Thomas, *et al., American Journal of Cardiology,* January, 1960.

[12] *Journal of the American Dietetic Association,* January, 1966.

Chapter 7

[1] P. J. Holloway, *et al., British Dental Journal,* May 6, 1958.

[2] Georg Lányi, M.D., "Raw Juices Instead of Drugs," *Tidskrift För Hälsa,* June, 1967.

[3] Lányi, "Raw Juices Instead of Drugs."

[4] Lányi, "Raw Juices Instead of Drugs."

Chapter 8

[1] A. Lwoff and M. Lwoff, Ann. Inst., Pasteur, September, 1961.

[2] Dr. Karl-Otto Aly, "Cancer Defeated by Body's Own Defenses," *Tidskrift För Hälsa,* September 9, 1965.

[3] Aly, "Cancer Defeated."

[4] Arne Timonen, "It Is Cold That Heals," *Tidskrift För Hälsa,* March, 1965.

[5] Harry F. Dietrich, M.D., *Dallas Morning News,* December 3, 1956.

Chapter 9

[1] Dr. L.-E. Essen, *Vidi Nova,* No. 1, 1964–65, p. 22. "The more extensive the chemical treatment—the less possibility for recovery."

[2] Adelle Davis, *Let's Get Well,* Harcourt, Brace & World, New York, 1965.

[3] *Proceedings of the Royal Society of Medicine,* Vol. XXX.

Chapter 10

[1] *New Physician,* May, 1964.

[2] *Lancet,* British Medical Journal, July 4, 1964.

[3] *Lancet,* December 17, 1966.

[4] *Tidskrift För Hälsa,* February 2, 1966.

[5] B. P. Sandler, M.D., *How to Prevent Heart Attacks,* Lee Foundation for Nutrition Research, 2023 West Wisconsin Ave., Milwaukee, Wisc.

[6] *Tidskrift För Hälsa,* February, 1966.

[7] *Tidskrift För Hälsa,* February, 1966.

[8] Sandler, *How to Prevent Heart Attacks.*

[9] Sandler. See also A. L. Myaknikov, *Circulation,* 17:99, 1958, and *Encyclopedia for Healthful Living,* Rodale Books, Inc., 1960.

[10] E. T. Gale, *et al., Geriatrics,* 8, 1953.

[11] *Encyclopedia for Healthful Living,* Rodale Books, Inc., 1960.

[12] W. J. McCormick, "Coronary Thrombosis: A New Concept of Mechanism and Etiology," *Clinical Medicine,* Vol. 4:7, 1957.

[13] *Canadian Medical Association Journal,* Vol. 44, 1941, p. 114.

[14] I. A. Miasnikov, *Terapevtichevskij Arkiv,* Vol. 28, 1956, p. 59. See also *Prevention,* February, 1967.

[15] *Polish Medical Journal,* Vol. 4, No. 6, 1965.

[16] L. M. Morrison, *et al., Proceedings of the Society of Biology and Medicine,* 73:37–38, 1950.

[17] Gilbert Dalldorf, M.D., *et al., The Avitaminoses,* Williams & Wilkins Co.

[18] P. A. Owren, *Lancet,* 2, 975, 1964.

[19] P. Prioreschi, *Canadian Medical Association Journal,* April 29, 1967.

[20] D. Kritchensky, *American Journal of Clinical Nutrition,* 10, 1962.

[21] W. A. Thomas, *et al., American Journal of Cardiology,* January, 1960.

Chapter 11

[1] Arnold DeVries, *Therapeutic Fasting,* Chandler Book Co., 1963.

[2] DeVries, *Therapeutic Fasting.*

[3] Y. Nishizawa, *et al., Journal of Vitaminology,* 3, 1957.

[4] "Vitamin P—Its Properties and Its Uses," National Science Foundation of the Department of Agriculture, 1963.

[5] F. G. Piotrowski, *Praxis,* July 1, 1948.

[6] Adelle Davis, *Let's Get Well,* Harcourt, Brace & World, New York, 1965.

Chapter 12

[1] Ebba Waerland, *Naturläkekonstens Bok,* Ny Nords Förlag, Sweden, 1961, and Are Waerland, *Health Is Your Birthright,* Humata Publishers, Bern, Switzerland.

[2] *New England Journal of Medicine,* Vol. 246, 1952, p. 721.

[3] *Science Newsletter,* July 4, 1953.

[4] *Acta Geographica,* 17, No. 4, 1963.

[5] K. Eckel and W. Lutz, *Vienna Clinical Weekly,* 73:493, 1961.

[6] E. M. Abrahamson, M. D., *Body, Mind and Sugar,* Holt, Rinehart & Winston, New York, 1951.

[7] Dr. Joseph Evers, *The Changed Aspects of Diseases* and *Directions for Treatment of Multiple Sclerosis,* Karl F. Haug Publishers, Ulm/Donau, West Germany, 1964.

[8] Ebba Waerland, *Naturläkekonstens Bok.*

[9] Are Waerland, *Health Is Your Birthright.*

[10] Adella Davis, *Let's Get Well,* Harcourt, Brace & World, New York, 1965.

Chapter 13

[1] "Läkartidningen," *Swedish Medical Journal,* 63, 45. 4292, 1966.

[2] *Medical World News,* March 26, 1965.

[3] *Journal of Vitaminology,* 11, 1–8, 1965.

[4] *Acta-Dermato-Venereologica,* 35–334, 1955.

Chapter 14

[1] L. E. Essén, "Pollen Som Läkemedel, *Vita Nova,* Sweden.

[2] Essén, "Pollen Som Läkemedel."

[3] *Life and Health,* March, 1959.

[4] Essén, "Pollen Som Läkemedel."

[5] *The Golden Pollen,* Yakima Bindery & Printing Co., Yakima, Wash., 1960.

[6] Pearson, *et al., Proceedings of the Society of Experimental Biology and Medicine,* Vol. 48, 1941, p. 415.

[7] *Acta Facultatis Pharmaceuticae Bohemoslovenicae,* Vol. X, 1965.

[8] P. Rovesti, Ref. Congr. XII, Lucerne, 1959.

[9] *Cancer Research,* 20, 503, 1960.

[10] *Journal of Pediatrics,* October, 1941.

Chapter 15

[1] "Aging, Atherosclerosis and Ascorbic Acid Metabolism," *The Journal of the American Geriatrics Society*, December, 1966.

[2] F. Verzer, "Report to the International Congress on Vitamin E," 1955.

Index

I

Infectious diseases, 95
Insecticides, 20, 21
Insomnia, 98
International Society for Research on Nutrition and Vital Substances, 79, 189–191, 198
Intestinal enzymes, 46–48

J

Jarvis, Dr. D. C., 178
Jonsson, Professor Gösta, 172
Journal of American Dietetic Association, 20
Journal of Gerontology, 176
Juice, 34–35
Juice fasts, 40–41
Juices, raw fruit and vegetable:
  diseases treated, 95–98
    blood and heart, 96
    blood pressure, 96
    diabetes, 97–98
    infectious, 95
    kidney disorders, 98
    leg ulcers, 96–97
    nervousness and insomnia, 98
    obesity, 97
    rheumatic, 97
    skin, 98
    stomach disorders, 95–96
  do-it-yourself treatment, 98–99
  juice—food or medicine, 90–91
  therapy, 91–94
    minerals, 92–93
    trace elements, 93
    vitamins, enzymes, coloring substances, etc., 93–94

K

Kasha, 202
Kefir, homemade, 205
Kellogg, Dr. Harvey, 139
Kelvin, Dr. John, 158
Kessler, Dr., 155
Kidney disorders, 98
Kneipp, Pastor, 56, 58
Kresanek, Dr. Jaroslav, 176
Kruska:
  uncooked quick, 201
  Waerland five-grain, 201
Kuratsune, Dr. M., 79
Kurorts sitz baths, 59

L

Lactase, 47
Lactic acid, 172
Lana, Risto, 34
Lányi, Dr. Georg, 91
Leander, Dr. Gösta, 172

Leaven, 49
Leg ulcers, 96–97
Lemon, Dr. Frank R., 85
Lepeshinskaya, Dr. Olga, 186
Let's Get Well, 154, 195
Life, Age and Longevity, 186
"Life force," 43–44
Lindlahr, Dr. Henry, 61
Lipase, 46
Liquid diet, 38
Liver and gallbladder, 95
"Living" water, 58–59
Low-animal-protein diet:
  empirical evidence, 82–86
    Bulgarians, 84–85
    Hunzakuts, 83
    Russians, 84
    Seventh-Day Adventists, 85–86
    Yemenites, 83–84
  fads and fallacies, 78–81
  fault with high-protein diet, 81–82
  high-protein myth, 76
  how much protein, 76–77
  how to plan, 87–88
  summary, 86–87
Low blood pressure, 96
Löyly, 104, 105
Lunch, 68
Lutz, Dr., 151
Lwoff, Dr. A., 100, 101

M

McCarrison, Sir Robert, 83
McCays, Dr. C. M., 126
McCormick, Dr. W. J., 107, 131
Macrobiotics, 188–191
Malnutrition, 19–20
Maltose, 45
Marches, fast, 28–31
Marshall, John, 81
Mayer, Dr. Adolph, 32
Mehren, George L., 20
Mesotrophy, 189
Metchnikoff, Dr. Ilja, 183, 184
Migraine, 71
Milk, 195
Milk, homemade soured, 204
Millet cereal, 202
Mineral waters, 52–64 (*see also Water*)
Moisteners, 20
Molino cereal, 202–203
Multiple sclerosis:
  advice to sufferers, 154
  causes, 149–150
  diet, 150–151
  Drs. Eckel and Lutz experiment, 151
  Evers diet therapy, 152–153
  vitamin F deficiency, 151
  Waerland therapy, 153–154

BLUEPRINTS FOR BETTER HEALTH

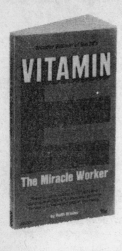

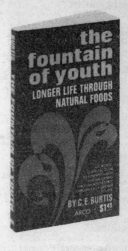

VITAMIN E—
THE MIRACLE WORKER

Ruth Winter

A simple, scientifically sound and comprehensive book that presents all the facts regarding the superb properties and marvelous potential of Vitamin E. Ruth Winter, a respected medical writer, examines the many claims and counter claims made for this extraordinary vitamin and reveals its reported usefullness in fighting infertility, ulcers and arthritis, its importance in preventing blood clots, its effectiveness against heart disease, cancer in animals and its significant role in retarding the aging process. Essential reading for everyone concerned about their own health and the health of their loved ones.   95¢

THE FOUNTAIN OF YOUTH

C.E. Burtis

A thorough guide to renewed vigor and well-being through wholesome organically grown foods, combined with a startling, fully documented expose of the adulterants and destructive processing that poison much of our daily fare. Based on a lifetime of research and experimentation in the field of nutrition, Mr. Burtis' book shows exactly how wholesome natural foods can bring renewed youth, vitality, fitness and the priceless gift of a longer life. Here are menus of easy-to-prepare health foods and eating methods that assure the best digestion and fullest use of a food's nourishing qualities as well as a discussion of dangerous foods. $1.45

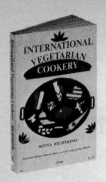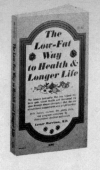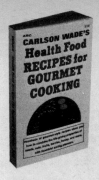

THE LOW-FAT WAY TO HEALTH AND LONGER LIFE

Lester Morrison, M.D.

The famous best-seller that has helped millions gain robust health
and increased life span through simple changes in diet, the use
of nutritional supplements and weight control. With menus, recipes,
life-giving diets, and programs endorsed by distinguished medical
authorities.   **$1.65**

CARLSON WADE'S HEALTH FOOD RECIPES FOR
GOURMET COOKING   Carlson Wade

Hundreds of recipes for preparing natural health foods—gourmet
style—for healthful eating pleasure. The secret of youthful energy
and vitality is in the magical powers of vitamins, minerals, enzymes, protein, and other life-giving elements found in **natural
foods.** In this new book, noted nutrition expert Carlson Wade
shows you how you can make delicious meals prepared with pure,
natural foods; seeds, nuts, berries, whole grains, honey, fruits,
fish and more.   **$1.65**

INTERNATIONAL VEGETARIAN COOKERY

Sonya Richmond

This book proves that vegetarian cookery, far from being dull and
difficult to prepare, can open up completely new and delightful
vistas of haute cuisine. Miss Richmond, who has traveled throughout the world, has arranged the book alphabetically according to
countries, starting with Austria and going through to the United
States. She gives recipes for each country's most characteristic
vegetarian dishes and lists that country's outstanding cheeses.

Clothbound: $3.75
Paperbound: $1.95

"THE MORE NATURAL OUR FOOD THE BETTER OUR HEALTH"

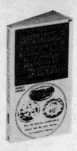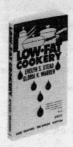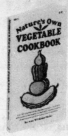

SOYBEAN (PROTEIN) RECIPE IDEAS
Nancy Snider

As a major source of protein soybeans are a nutritious and endlessly versatile food. Here are over 100 unusual and delicious recipes that take the zesty soybean from breakfast to dinner in a fabulous cookbook by a noted home economist and food editor. Scores of diet and dollar stretching recipes—all easy to prepare and serve—and all featuring soy protein—soy stroganoff, meat loaf, soy breakfast items, soups, entrees, side dishes, sandwiches, breads, desserts, much more. Includes menu ideas and tips on cooking with soy.

Illustrated, 95¢

LOW-FAT COOKERY
Evelyn S. Stead and Gloria K. Warren

Here finally is the perfect cookbook for a calorie-conscious, health-happy age. Incorporating more than 250 delicious, easy-to-follow recipes, **Low-Fat Cookery** puts the fun into dietetic cooking—and even more imporant, dietetic eating. Imagine delicious low-fat recipes for baked lasagna, fruitcake, bleu-cheese dressing, butterscotch sauce and lobster newburg. Included are invaluable aids to dietetic cooking with an easy-to-remember summary of the basic points of low-fat cookery, how to modify any recipe to obtain a low-fat content, information about new food products to enrich and diversify a low-fat diet, and a helpful discussion of special diets such as restricted sodium and unsaturated vegetable oil plans. $1.45

NATURE'S OWN VEGETABLE COOKBOOK
Ann Williams-Heller

Over 350 mouthwatering vegetable recipes—complete with practical information on the buying, storing, cooking, seasoning and nutritional value of each vegetable. With this cookbook, noted nutritionist Ann Williams-Heller has opened the door to an entirely new culinary world. She brings her cooking genius to bear on every available vegetable—in main dishes, casseroles, salads, soups and their countless variations. Also included are recipes for sauces and salad dressings as well as nutrition charts that show the vitamin and mineral content of each vegetable. $1.45

READ YOUR WAY TO BETTER HEALTH